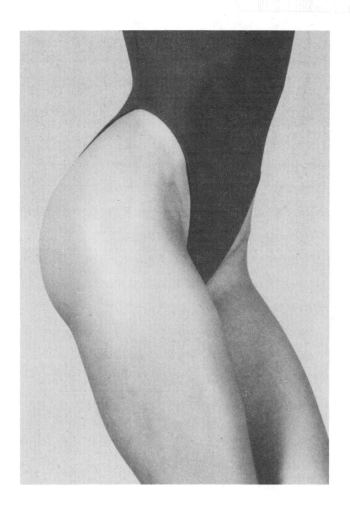

OTHER BOOKS OF INTEREST
• • •

By Ellington Darden, Ph.D.

The Nautilus Diet

The Six-Week Fat-to-Muscle Makeover

The Nautilus Book (Revised Edition)

The Nautilus Bodybuilding Book (Revised Edition)

New High-Intensity Bodybuilding

100 High-Intensity Ways to Improve Your Bodybuilding

The Athlete's Guide to Sports Medicine

Nutrition for Athletes

The Nautilus Nutrition Book

The Nautilus Woman (Revised Edition)

How to Lose Body Fat

32 Days to a 32-Inch Waist

For a free catalog of Dr. Darden's fitness books, please send a self-addressed, stamped envelope to Nautilus Sports/Medical Industries, P.O. Box 160, Independence, VA 24348.

HOT HIPS
&
FABULOUS THIGHS

Ellington Darden, Ph.D.

TAYLOR PUBLISHING COMPANY
Dallas, Texas

Book Designed by Deborah Jackson-Jones

Published by Taylor Publishing Company
    1550 West Mockingbird Lane
    Dallas, Texas 75235

Library of Congress Cataloging-in-Publication Data

Darden, Ellington, 1943–
    Hot hips and fabulous thighs / Ellington Darden.
        p. cm.
    ISBN 0-87833-733-4 : $9.95
    1. Reducing exercises.   2. Weight lifting.   3. Low-calorie diet.
    4. Exercise for women.   I. Title.   II. Title: Hot hips and fabulous
    thighs.
    RA781.6.D374   1991
    646.7'5—dc20   90-20566
                                                                        CIP

Printed in the United States of America

10 9 8 7 6 5

ACKNOWLEDGMENTS

Many people deserve thanks for their contributions to this book.

Brenda Hutchins planned the menus, recipes, and shopping lists.

Ken Hutchins and Kirk Wilder took the before-and-after photographs. Kenn Thorpe snapped the photo on page viii.

Dan Howard inputted my handwritten pages into his word processor and made the necessary revisions.

Carole Burrow, Connie May, and Darcy Wyler read the manuscript and offered many valuable suggestions.

Alicia Tannery took the front cover photograph as well as the exercise photographs.

Brenda Smedley, Raney Grasso, and Carol Kentzel displayed their great-looking hips and thighs for the cover.

Brenda Smedley and Amy Floyd demonstrated the exercise routines in Chapters 23 and 24.

Raney Grasso and Brenda Smedley helped organize the freehand exercise routines. They also trained many of the women featured in the book.

Special appreciation goes to the Exchange Athletic Club, the Uptowner Athletic Club, the Lincoln Fitness Center, and to all the women who participated in the research for this project.

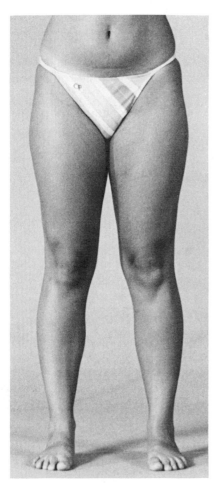 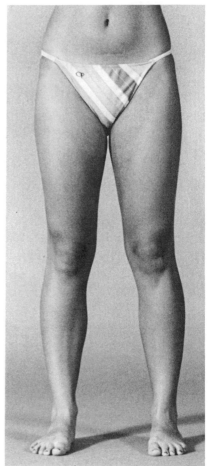

Before   **After**

To get Hot Hips and Fabulous Thighs, Dawn Prochaska **LOST** 19 ³/₄ pounds of fat and **RESHAPED** her body with 3 ¹/₂ pounds of muscle. She also **TRIMMED** 3 ¹/₄ inches off her waist, 3 ¹/₂ inches off her hips, and 5 inches off her upper thighs.

CONTENTS

—— •••——

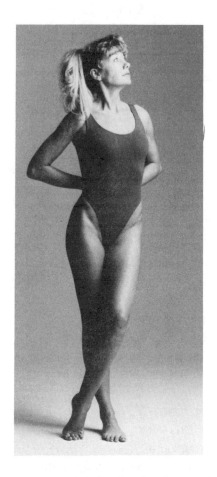

With the exercise plan in this book, Carol Kentzel, age 35, added 4 1/4 pounds of figure-firming muscle to her arms and lower body.

···**1**···
Hot and Fabulous: The Details

$\vdots$

You can get the great hips and thighs you've always wanted by losing up to:

- 4 inches off your hips
- 5 inches off your thighs
- 20 pounds of body fat

and by adding 4 pounds of figure-shaping muscle. Doing so, in fact, takes only six weeks.

Want proof? The before-and-after photographs throughout this book are of women who have been through the recommended program.

Yes, you can drastically change the size and shape of your lower body. Hot Hips and Fabulous Thighs can be yours.

··● THE *HOT* AND THE *FABULOUS*

Exactly what are Hot Hips and Fabulous Thighs?

They are hips and thighs you can be proud of. More specifically, Hot Hips are firm, tight, and shapely buttocks. Fabulous Thighs are long, lean, and strong from all angles: front, back, and sides.

Not only will you see significant improvement in the appearance and condition of your hips and thighs after just six weeks of the program, but you'll notice reshaping in your waist and upper body as well. Plus, you'll welcome the guidelines on food, nutrition, cooking, exercise physiology, self-image, water, and tanning.

By the end of this program, you'll be well-equipped in both body and mind. First, a little background on the project will prove helpful.

1

••• DEVELOPING THE CONCEPT

"Women everywhere want to lose fat from their hips and thighs," Alicia Tannery said to me as we walked up Fifth Avenue in New York City.

"You're right," I concurred as I eyed the passing parade of women in their designer clothes. "I'd sure like to come up with an intriguing title for a new diet and exercise program for women. Something more exciting than *The Hip and Thigh Diet*. Perhaps, one I could use in conjunction with 32/32."

32/32 was an executive fitness project (and *32 Days to a 32-Inch Waist* the resulting book) that I worked on in 1988 and 1989. Several hundred men were supervised through the 32-day plan in three large fitness centers in Dallas with great success. Alicia's father, Zack, was one of the subjects who did the best. He had lost 28 1/2 pounds of fat.

As a result, Zack turned into one of the program's biggest supporters. He recruited his wife, daughter (Alicia), son, daughter-in-law, and at least six friends.

I'd tell Zack and the women he recruited that the 32/32 program was designed for men who desired a 32-inch waist. The concept should still work for women, Zack would insist. He was right to a certain extent. Telling women that they should *not* get involved wasn't the answer.

I realized that what I wanted—and what thousands of women wanted—was a diet plan specific to women's problems. Men are primarily concerned about their waists. Women think *hips* and *thighs*.

••• THE ATTENTION-GETTER

"I need an attention-getter, something that will pique a woman's interest just by reading the title," I said to Alicia as we continued our walk up Fifth Avenue. Alicia was enrolled in the photography department at New York University. I wanted her to meet Marty Moskof, who does the layout and design for many of my fitness books. Marty's office was on West 57th Street.

Halfway through our meeting with Marty, Alicia lit up with an energetic smile. "I've got an idea for the title. How about *Hot Hips and Fabulous Thighs?*"

"Say no more," said Marty. "*Hot Hips and Fabulous Thighs* says it all. That's what women want."

"It's the ideal attention-getter and the perfect title for my new research project and book," I said as we nodded in agreement.

All I needed at this point was a diet and exercise plan that delivered that promise. That would be relatively easy, since I already had an understanding and application of the basics from my previous programs.

•• REQUIREMENTS AND RESEARCH

The next day I flew back to Dallas and went to work on the new project. My goal was a six-week diet that provided from 1,400 to 1,000 calories a day—and also included frozen dinners. Certain frozen dinners, which are available at all supermarkets, are nutritious and easy to prepare. Busy people love them because they take the hassle out of the evening meal. At the same time, it's important for dieters to learn how to weigh and measure food, count calories accurately, and cook some foods from scratch.

The Hot Hips and Fabulous Thighs diet needed to do all of the above, as well as provide ample variety for most meals.

Of equal importance was the exercise routine. The exercise would be performed on Nautilus equipment, or with freehand movements using body weight as resistance.

I've designed many successful courses employing Nautilus, barbells, and dumbbells. I had not experimented extensively with freehand floor exercises that are so popular with women today. I predicted that if properly performed, using slow movements and sustained contractions, it would produce dramatic bodyshaping results.

For several months I tested, retested, and fine-tuned the diet and exercises. When I thought the course was sound, I took it to the Exchange Athletic Club in downtown Dallas. I've conducted much research at this club, since it has a large membership of both men and women who are receptive to new programs.

One problem I faced, however, made me a bit hesitant. It was almost November, which meant the program would have to run through Thanksgiving and well into December. Because of the holiday festivities, November and December are generally the worst months of the year to begin a diet. January and February, conversely, are usually the best months.

I decided to announce the program immediately, start it within a week, and see what would happen.

Initially, I worried that I might not have enough participants for even one research group. Surprisingly, twice as many women as I needed showed up for the introductory meeting, and I signed up enough subjects for two groups.

I realized then the power behind the concept of *Hot* Hips and *Fabulous* Thighs.

Since that time more than 100 women have been through the course. They've been tested and trained in Orlando, Florida; Long Island, New York; and Dallas, Texas.

••• MOVE TO ACTION

Results have been stunning. You can lose inches and pounds quickly . . . in all the right places.

Hot Hips and Fabulous Thighs are only a few weeks away. Sounds exciting, doesn't it?

Let's get started!

···2···

Quiz Yourself

.

"How is this diet different?" is one of the first questions typically asked about a new diet.

"How can I succeed using this diet plan when all the others I've tried have failed?" is usually the next query, followed by: "Will this program get rid of the fat around my hips and thighs?"

To help answer these questions, here are 15 true-or-false statements about diet and exercise. Please read each one carefully before circling your choice.

··● TRUE OR FALSE

T	F	1.	The problem is that you need to lose weight—10, 15, 20, or more pounds.
T	F	2.	In a six-week diet program, general guidelines are more important than specific rules.
T	F	3.	It's essential to limit your consumption of carbohydrate-rich foods, such as bread, rice, and potatoes.
T	F	4.	A sound fat-loss diet reduces your calories from fat to from 10–15 percent of your total calories per day.

5

T   F   5. Skipping a meal occasionally is a great way to lose fat.

T   F   6. Snacks are taboo on a lower-calorie diet.

T   F   7. The idea that *diets don't work* is correct.

T   F   8. To maximize fat loss, it is important to exercise every day.

T   F   9. Stretching movements are the cornerstone of a successful fat-loss plan.

T   F   10. Aerobic exercise is necessary for maximum fat loss.

T   F   11. Running is a fantastic exercise for spot reducing your lower body.

T   F   12. Fast exercise is more productive than slow exercise for shaping your legs.

T   F   13. Building the muscles of your hips and thighs will make your legs look bigger and is of little value in reducing the fatty deposits in those areas.

T   F   14. For best results when dieting you should drink 6–8 glasses of water each day.

T   F   15. Cellulite is *fat-gone-wrong* that accumulates on your hips and thighs.

••• THE FACTS ABOUT DIETING AND EXERCISING

How many of these statements do you consider true? Most women who have been on diets believe at least half of them are valid.

The correct answer is that *all of them are false.*

If you believe in the truth of even *one* of the statements, that belief itself could well be responsible for the failure of all your previous dieting and exercising efforts.

For example, in statement #1, if you think you need to lose 15 pounds, then several concepts deserve attention.

First, losing weight is largely a misnomer. Most women need to lose *fat* much more than they need to lose *weight*. Second, the solution to the problem not only requires fat loss but positive changes in your lifestyle. Third, *permanent* fat loss should be your goal. Permanent fat loss involves understanding and applying several easy-to-learn physical, psychological, and social factors. A complete discussion of these factors follows in Chapters 4, 9, and 10.

Statement #2, general versus specific guidelines, merits several chapters. Successful dieters I've worked with over the years thrive on specificity much more than generality.

If you circled "T" after reading statements #3–#7, your attitude virtually guaranteed that all your previous dieting efforts would fail. But don't get too depressed. Similar misconceptions are implicit in nine out of ten dieting books. Chapter 9 will set the record straight.

Proper exercise is a key to fat loss. Exercise, however, must be clearly defined and applied or it can cause more harm than good. It comes as no surprise that most women, as well as physicians, regard statements #8–#13 on exercise as true. You'll become intimately associated with proper exercise in Chapters 11, 12, 23, and 24.

The importance of drinking water in dieting and exercising has recently drawn some attention. The standard recommendation is to consume from 6–8 glasses a day. In my research, though, I've found that you'll get much better results by tripling that amount. You'll learn why in Chapter 10.

The last statement, cellulite is fat-gone-wrong, is thought to be true by most women. Scientifically, there is no such thing as cellulite. It is not a special type of fat that has gone wrong. It is simply regular fat that has been deposited in thick layers around hips and thighs of most overfat women. Often this thick layering becomes dimpled and rippled.

The cure for the cellulite look, and the solution to those lumps and bumps, is the program you are holding in your hands: *Hot Hips and Fabulous Thighs.*

••• FROM FALSE TO TRUE

With the program in this book, you'll gradually change your false beliefs about dieting and exercising to tried-and-true habits. Why? Because you'll see tangible proof in your own body:

- firm, tight, and shapely buttocks
- long, lean, and strong thighs

In the next chapter you'll meet some women who achieved their goal of Hot Hips and Fabulous Thighs.

··· 3 ···
Look at My
Hips and Thighs

Few women are ever completely happy with the way they look. The most disliked body part, according to a *Family Circle* (February 1, 1990) questionnaire, is the hips/buttocks area. The thighs rank a close second.

"If only my hips matched the rest of me," fret most of these women. "If only I could firm and tighten my thunder thighs," echo almost as many.

Hips and thighs: Fat and Flabby, or Hot and Fabulous? The choice is up to you.

Women in this chapter chose the latter. You'll be motivated by looking at their before-and-after pictures.

*"**I**'m so pleased with my new body. I now know there's a difference between looking good and looking great. It's definitely worth the hard work."*

SHERRI BARNHART
—————————— •••• ——————————

age: 25
height: 5'6"

LOST 10¼ pounds of fat, **RESHAPED** her body by adding 2 pounds of muscle, and **TRIMMED** 2 inches off her waist, 2¼ inches off her hips, and 2 inches off her upper thighs in six weeks.

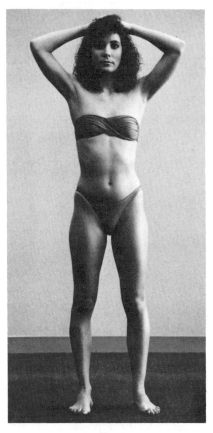
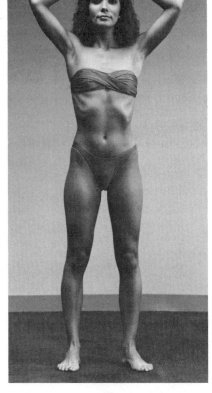

Before   **After**

*"**A**fter having a baby last year, I just couldn't seem to get back into shape. I felt unattractive and tired all the time.*

"Now, I feel good about myself. My work performance has improved. I have more energy. I feel younger."

PAM SMITH
•••

age: 28
height: 5'6"

LOST 15 pounds of fat, **RESHAPED** her body by adding 2½ pounds of muscle, and **TRIMMED** 3⅞ inches off her waist, 2⅜ inches off her hips, and 3¼ inches off her upper thighs in six weeks.

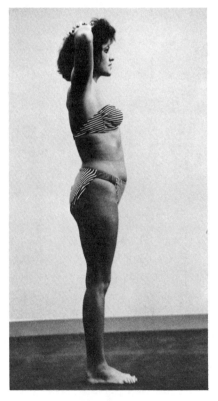 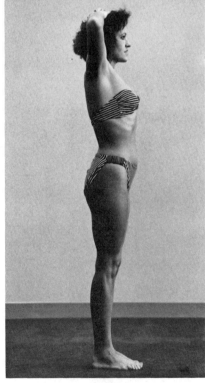

Before　　　　　　　　　　　　　**After**

*"**M**y hips were out of proportion to my upper body. Now, I like the way my hips look, especially from the back."*

KATHLEEN BERTHOLD
— • • • —

age: 29
height: 5'8"

LOST 11 pounds of fat, **RESHAPED** her body by adding 1 pound of muscle, and **TRIMMED** 2 1/4 inches off her waist, 2 1/4 inches off her hips, and 3 1/4 inches off her upper thighs in six weeks.

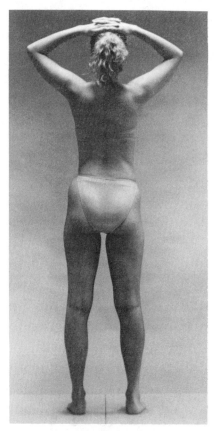 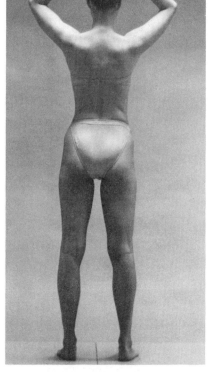

Before   **After**

*"**M**y hips and thighs are dramatically reshaped. I feel so much better about myself. With the program, I turned self-doubt into self-assurance."*

BRIDGET KLEINE
• • •
age: 29
height: 5'5 1/2"

LOST 18 1/2 pounds of fat, **RESHAPED** her body by adding 1 pound of muscle, and **TRIMMED** 3 3/4 inches off her waist, 2 inches off her hips, and 3 1/2 inches off her upper thighs in six weeks.

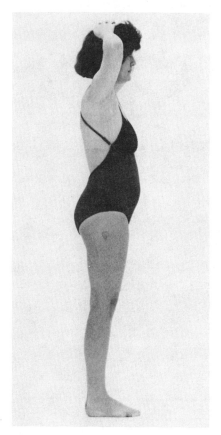
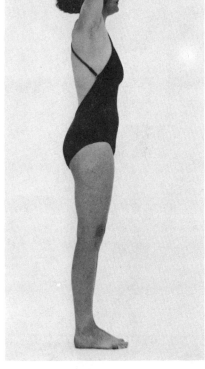

Before   **After**

"I love to wear shorts during the summer. As a result of the program, I've never received so many compliments about the appearance of my hips and thighs. I know you can't stop the aging process, but you can certainly forestall it."

CAROL JACKSON
•••

age: 28

height: 5'5 ½"

LOST 17 pounds of fat, **RESHAPED** her body by adding 2 pounds of muscle, and **TRIMMED** 4 inches off her waist, 2 ¾ inches off her hips, and 4 inches off her upper thighs in six weeks.

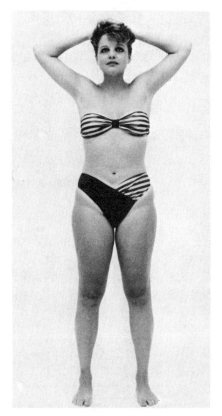
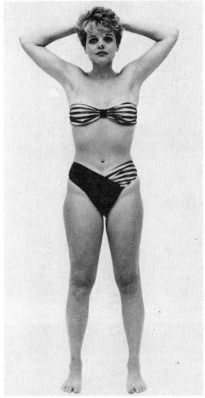

Before   **After**

··· 4 ···

Muscle/Fat Ratio

Weighing on the bathroom scales is a daily ritual for most women.

How much do you weigh?

There is a prevalent belief that appearance and well-being depend on body weight.

Your body weight and the standard height-weight comparisons are simply a rough estimate of the shape, condition, and appearance of your figure. To be more meaningful, your body weight must be broken down into four components.

··· COMPONENTS OF BODY WEIGHT

The four major components of your body are:

- Bone
- Organs
- Muscle
- Fat

Muscle and fat are those most critical to this discussion and most subject to significant modification through diet and exercise.

Much of the challenge of achieving Hot Hips and Fabulous Thighs centers around an understanding of muscle and fat, or more specifically, optimizing your muscle-to-fat ratio.

••• THE AVERAGE WOMAN

Over the past five years, I've done body composition measurements on over 1,000 women. In addition I've talked with and observed the figure problems of thousands more. The following chart is representative of the average woman that I've worked with. Let's follow her body composition from age 14 to 50.

MUSCLE/FAT RATIO CHANGES
•••
In Average Woman As She Ages

Age:	14	20	30	40	50
Body Weight (Pounds)	120	126	136	146	156
Muscle (Pounds)	48	45	40	35	30
Fat (Pounds)	20	29	44	59	74
Muscle/Fat Ratio	2.4/1	1.55/1	1/1.1	1/1.69	1/2.47
Percent Body Fat	16.7	23.0	32.4	40.4	47.4

Between the ages of 14–50, the average woman loses .5 pounds of muscle per year and gains 1.5 pounds of fat per year.

My measurements and observations show that the average woman is generally at her peak physically at age 14. At a height of 5 feet 4 inches and a body weight of 120 pounds, her muscle weighs 48 pounds and her fat weighs 20 pounds. Her muscle/fat ratio is 48/20 or 2.4/1. In other words, she has 2.4 pounds of muscle for each pound of fat. Because of this high ratio of muscle to fat, her body is firm, hard, and well defined.

With each passing year, however, she loses .5 pounds of muscle and gains 1.5 pounds of fat. The specifics are listed in the chart.

••• AGE 50

At age 50 she weighs 156 pounds, which is a gain of 36 pounds of body weight since age 14. More specifically, her muscle has decreased by 18 pounds and her fat has increased by 54 pounds. Her muscle/fat ratio has changed from 2.4/1 to 1/2.47, which is a complete reversal. Furthermore, her percentage of body fat goes from 16.7 to 47.4—a 284 percent increase.

What causes this influx of fat and gradual loss of muscle? The primary reasons are too many dietary calories, faulty eating habits, lack of proper exercise, a reduced metabolic rate, pregnancy and childbirth, overstress, and the natural aging process.

••• MORE MUSCLE, LESS FAT

To correct her figure problems, the average woman in her 20s, 30s, 40s, or 50s requires more muscle and less fat. The average woman needs what the Hot Hips and Fabulous Thighs program has to offer.

What about you? Are you similar to the average woman described in this chapter? Isn't it time you corrected the situation?

All of the causative factors listed in the last section, with the exception of the aging process, are subject to your control. With discipline, patience, and the guidelines presented in this book, you can successfully lose fat and build muscle at the same time. Doing so will have a significant effect on your muscle/fat ratio and an enormous effect on the appearance of your hips and thighs.

···5···
Why Women Store Fat Around Their Hips and Thighs
⦂

Unfortunately, women and men do *not* live in an equal world when it concerns the amount and the concentration of body fat.

Females mature fatter than males. Men, with their greater height and larger muscles and bones, are heavier. But when it comes to the amount of body weight composed of adipose tissue, women are the fatter sex. The average woman has at least two times as much fat around her hips and thighs as does the average man.

Why do women have more fat than men and, in particular, thicker layers around their hips and thighs? The answer is those wonderful hormones. Hormones are also the reason that most women have a much harder time losing fat than do men.

To understand, combat, and conquer the situation requires a basic knowledge of four related factors.

••● PUBERTY

There is minimal difference in the body fat levels between the two sexes in childhood. At puberty, however, girls begin putting on fat and boys start putting on muscle. A girl must have approximately 15 to 20 percent of her weight as fat before she can start to menstruate.

A low percentage of body fat is the reason some girls who are very athletic, such as gymnasts, ballerinas, and runners, frequently begin menstruating several years later than their more sedentary peers. Oftentimes their activity levels must be reduced to allow for normal fat gain, which then kicks into action their hormones and brings about regular menstrual cycles.

18

••• MENSTRUATION

Both men and women produce hormones that make them characteristically male or female. For women, the two main hormones are estrogen and progesterone. Both can contribute to fatness.

The interacting rise and fall of estrogen and progesterone regulate a woman's menstrual cycle. The entire cycle, from ovulation to menstruation to ovulation, takes from 25 to 32 days.

The same estrogen that is involved in your menstrual cycle also causes you to deposit fat in your breasts, hips, buttocks, and thighs. It does this by chemically stimulating fat cells in those areas to store fat.

Progesterone jumps in by affecting your appetite and mood. It makes you hungrier during the second half of the menstrual cycle and is also responsible for the ravenous appetite that many women have during pregnancy. Progesterone can also make you feel sluggish, sleepy, and less inclined to exercise.

Both estrogen and certain by-products of progesterone cause you to retain fluid. This can make your rings and shoes feel tight during the few days just before your period begins, which is often referred to as premenstrual syndrome. As you are probably aware, it's common to gain from 3 to 5 pounds and to feel uncomfortable at this time of the month. Fortunately, when the estrogen and progesterone levels fall leading to menstruation, the excess fluid subsides, and the other uncomfortable sensations disappear as well.

••• BIRTH CONTROL PILLS

Birth control pills are still the most popular form of contraception in the United States. There are different types of pills, but the most popular is a combination of synthetic estrogen and progesterone.

The average woman who takes birth control pills gains approximately 3 to 5 pounds of body weight as a side effect and most of it is fat. These pills are fattening for the same reasons your body's natural estrogen and progesterone are. Fortunately, most of the pills used today contain much less estrogen and progesterone than the earlier pills. As a result, the newer birth control pills cause less weight gain.

••• PREGNANCY

There is no doubt about it—pregnancy is very fattening.

Research shows that the average weight gain from the beginning of the first trimester until the end of pregnancy is 27.5 pounds, of which about 20 percent is fat. Your progesterone levels stay high from the beginning of your pregnancy to the end. Instead of making you hungrier for a few days each month, this hormone stimulates your appetite continuously for the entire nine months.

Progesterone is not the real culprit, however, when it comes to weight gain during pregnancy. That distinction belongs to the fat cells.

Fat cells can multiply during periods of rapid growth, such as infancy and puberty. Men and women can also add fat cells any time they add weight quickly. But with pregnancy, women have a high risk for fat-cell increase that men never have to endure.

The number of fat cells you add depends on how much and how fast you gain fat. Further pregnancies can compound the process. Once a fat cell has been formed, it stays with you for the rest of your life, always demanding to be filled. This is the primary reason most of the fat gained during pregnancy tends to hang on so tenaciously, long after the baby has been born.

Wide, thick, and fleshy hips and buttocks also facilitate pregnancy and the birth process. A proportional amount of fat is usually deposited around the upper thighs. Women with natural tendencies toward these characteristics have an easier time giving birth than women with thin hips, flat buttocks, and lean thighs.

••• FATED TO BE FAT?

As I've explained, storing extra fat around the hips and thighs is intimately associated with menstruation, pregnancy, and reproduction. Such fatness is a fact of biological life and one that was programmed into the species long ago by nature. But why?

Because most of our ancestors lived in a time of snow and ice and they adapted by getting fatter. Lean people tended to die out, while the fat people tended to survive and reproduce.

Fat helped our ancestors keep warm, and it gave them a portable food supply when vegetation was absent and game was scarce. Over the centuries a genetic preference for fat was built into our makeup. Interestingly, an aesthetic preference went with it. Not only was fat necessary for life itself, fat also seemed beautiful.

We'll find out why in the next chapter, and we'll discuss how the fat-is-beautiful concept has changed over the last 70 years.

Before we do, the question: "Are women fated to be fat?" must be answered.

Most women do inherit a large number of fat cells around their hips and thighs for the reasons stated in this chapter. But regardless of the number, fat cells can shrink. You can lose significant pounds and inches from your lower body.

Depending on your genetics, however, you may have a harder time getting lean than does the average woman. If that's the case, you'll deal with the fact best by facing it head-on and realizing that you'll require extra time and effort to overcome it.

None of these drawbacks spell ultimate doom. If you want to have a lean body with great hips and thighs badly enough, and if you're willing to abandon the quick-and-easy answers and combat a difficult problem realistically, no roadblocks will stop you.

No! You are not fated to be fat.

You can have Hot Hips and Fabulous Thighs!

···6···

Beauty and Fat Through the Ages

•

Something is of value, generally speaking, if it contributes to survival and prosperity. If something is difficult to get, it becomes even more valuable.

It should be obvious that concepts of beauty are closely linked with the laws of economics. What people find valuable, they also tend to find beautiful.

Fat was appealing originally for two reasons. First, it had immense survival and reproductive value. Second, when fat people were scarce, being fat carried with it status, especially for women.

••• FEMALE STATUS

The division of labor among our Stone Age ancestors was simple. The men hunted and the women bore children. Agriculture did not exist.

The women could eat what little they could gather from the sparse vegetation. The men, however, controlled the majority of the food supply. What meat they didn't consume from a kill, they brought back to the cave to share with the women and children.

The leftovers went to the women the hunters found most attractive. Thus, the attractive women had the best chance to get fat, and fatness became a trait of sexiness and status. The practice was self-perpetuating: sexy women got fat, and fat women were considered sexy.

Fatness was also considered valuable and beautiful because it was associated with fertility. In the last chapter, we discussed that it takes a certain amount of body fat for a woman to conceive, bear, and nourish a child. The fatter women of the Stone Age had fewer miscarriages and stillbirths, and produced more and healthier babies, than their leaner friends.

Fertile females were prized. The fatter they were and the broader they were at the hips, the better. The rigors of life at that time allowed few women to survive to even 30 years of age. The period of breeding was brief, so children were at a premium.

••• LAW OF SUPPLY AND DEMAND

Why did the attraction for fatness continue to persist after the Stone Age?

Because the same law of supply and demand was still at work. What's scarce is valuable. Food, and fatness, remained relative rarities for a long time.

Even in the richest of ancient civilizations, comfort and plenty were available only to a few. The vast majority of people remained poor, surviving at sustenance level. Wars, plagues, floods, and famines were recurrences that disrupted whole populations. In short, humankind enjoyed very few plush times and many centuries of scarcity.

Only with the coming of the Industrial Revolution some 140 years ago did prosperity become moderately widespread, and only in advanced nations. Until then, most people worked very hard for very little, and few could afford getting fat.

So, the fat-is-beautiful concept rules when times are hard, and times have usually been hard. What happens, however, when times are easy?

••• EASY STREET

During times of prosperity, fat loses its survival value and its status. Fat becomes ugly. Lean becomes beautiful.

The American attitude toward feminine beauty began to shift in the early 1920s. The United States was enjoying exceptional prosperity. Technology was making giant strides. Old values and sexual role models were being questioned. The woman's suffrage movement was gaining momentum. The motion picture industry was beginning.

Women became more liberated. They bobbed their hair, shortened their skirts, and became more active. A slender figure seemed better proportioned for the shorter skirt, and better suited for activity.

Thus, a leaner, sometimes skinny, role model for the average American woman began to emerge. Today, thinness is still very much in vogue.

••• UGLY FAT

On average, however, we Americans are certainly not getting leaner. We are among the richest people in the world, among the fattest, and easily the most obsessed with losing weight.

For us, food is abundant and relatively cheap. Few people miss meals, and fewer fear starvation. We suffer not from undernutrition, but from overnutrition.

Fatness has now become common. No longer a symbol of status, being fat is now deemed dowdy and lower class. In simple terms, fat is no longer sexy. Fat is ugly.

••• REASONABLE AND REALISTIC

Despite the current trend, there's nothing innately ugly about fat. There are good reasons, however, to reduce your excess. Most of them center around health and longevity. For example, obesity complicates the following: high blood pressure, kidney disease, gall bladder disease, diabetes mellitus, osteoarthritis and gout, and breast and endometrial cancer. Reducing body fat decreases the probability of the occurrence of the above illnesses. Leaner bodies are healthier bodies.

Aesthetics, however, are also important. That's probably the reason you bought this book. How you look can certainly affect all kinds of social, psychological, and physiological factors. Be careful that you don't make yourself miserable dwelling on your failure to conform to the current standard of what's beautiful. Few women can ever look like the models they hold in high esteem.

Evaluate accurately your body fat level and your hip and thigh status. Then, set reasonable and realistic goals for yourself. Chapter 8 shows you how.

First let's take a close look at one of the most dreaded words in a woman's vocabulary: cellulite.

•• 7 ••

Cellulite: Combating Those Lumps and Bumps

Is your cellulite showing?

Would you like to smooth it away?

If so, then as I said in Chapter 2, *Hot Hips and Fabulous Thighs* is the program for you.

Although there is no such scientific term as cellulite, the condition to which the word refers does exist.

Most women have thick layers of fat directly under the skin on their upper thighs and buttocks. Cellulite is subcutaneous (beneath the skin) adipose tissue just like any common body fat. The dimpled effect is caused by the fibers of connective tissue in the area, which lose their elasticity with age. The overlying skin attached to these fibers then contracts. If the size of the encased fat cells does not shrink proportionately, a kind of overall dimpling occurs on the surface of the skin.

Before we discuss the specific cure for dimpled fat, let's briefly examine the origin of cellulite.

•• THE ORIGIN OF CELLULITE

The concept of cellulite, pronounced *cell-u-leet,* was introduced in the United States by Nicole Ronsard. In 1973, she wrote a best-selling book titled *Cellulite: Those Lumps, Bumps and Bulges You Couldn't Lose Before.*

Madame Ronsard, as she prefers to be called, notes in the book's introduction that she came across the word "cellulite" while she was studying in France. French beauty experts supposedly learned of cellulite from Swedish doctors over eighty years ago. More recently, according to Madame Ronsard, French scientists perfected a way to eliminate cellulite.

The French techniques were brought by Madame Ronsard to the United States, where she offered classes from her New York figure salon. Six years later, her book on the subject was published in both hardback and paperback editions. The paperback version is still available in most bookstores.

"Talk about cellulite! Well, I had it, from my lower back down to my mid-thighs. Now, those lumps and bumps have been smoothed away.

"The program has been a godsend. I'm elated with the results."

CARLA BINION
• • •

age: 30

height: 5'9 3/4"

LOST 18 3/4 pounds of fat, **RESHAPED** her body by adding 3 1/4 pounds of muscle, and **TRIMMED** 4 5/8 inches off her waist, 2 1/4 inches off her hips, and 5 1/8 inches off her upper thighs in twelve weeks.

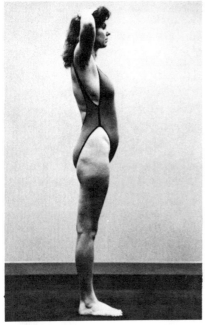
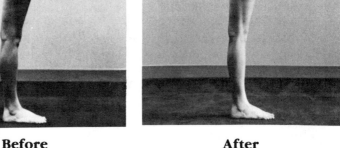

Before   **After**

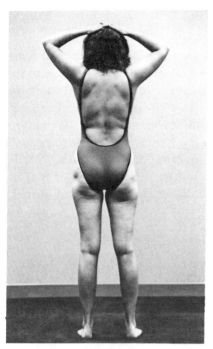 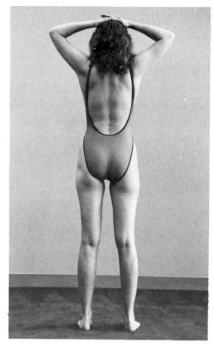

| **Before** | **After** |

According to Madame Ronsard, cellulite is not regular fat. "It is a gel-like substance made up of fat, water, and wastes trapped in bumpy, immovable pockets just beneath the skin. The pockets of *fat-gone-wrong* act like sponges that can absorb large amounts of water, blow up, and bulge out, resulting in ripples and flabbiness you see."

••• CELLULITE MISINFORMATION

Since Madame Ronsard believes that cellulite is not normal fat, she claims that the typical diet-and-exercise routines have no effect in removing it. What is needed, she says, is a six-part plan involving diet, elimination, breathing, exercise, massage, and relaxation. Since most cellulite information involves a variation of Ronsard's plan, a brief overview of each part will be helpful. (1) *Diet:* Avoid foods such as pork, bacon, macaroni, cheese, tuna, and bread, which she says leave toxic residues in the body. (2) *Proper elimi-nation:* Her elimination program consists of drinking six to eight glasses of water a day, consuming a glass of prune juice and a table-spoon of vegetable oil daily, taking a sauna bath twice a week, and having a dry friction rub with a loofah mitten after your daily shower. (3) *Breathing and oxygenation:* She recommends yoga deep-breathing exercises as a way to oxygenate the body and loosen harmful impurities from the lung tissue. (4) *Exercise:* A series of yoga and calisthenic-type exercises are to be performed for at least fifteen minutes each day, seven days a week. (5) *Massage:* Ronsard suggests that a woman devote from twenty to thirty minutes a day to kneading, knuckling, and wringing those cellulite-containing areas of the hips and thighs. (6) *Relaxation:* It is emphasized that when a woman learns to relax muscle properly, her circulation is improved and the release of toxic residues is encouraged.

Ronsard's six-part plan is not scientifically sound. Nor is it an efficient way for a woman to get rid of her fatty lumps and bulges.

••• THE REAL FACTS ABOUT CELLULITE

The truth about cellulite is as follows:

- Cellulite is nothing more than stored fat.

- The dimpling effect of the fat on the overlying skin is caused by a combination of overfatness, loss of muscular size and strength, and the natural aging of the connective tissue.

- All stored fat, regardless of its location, is hard to remove from the human body.

- Women store several times more fat on their hips and thighs than do men. Much of this is related to hormones and the ability to conceive children.

- Quick and easy solutions to removing dimpled fatty deposits are based on half-truths, myths, ignorance, and outright lies. They do not produce lasting results.

- Fat cannot be massaged, perspired, relaxed, soaked, flushed, compressed, or dissolved out of the human body.

••• THE CURE

The treatment for dimpled fatty deposits is a two-fold approach.

- You must reduce the size of the fat cells by dieting.
- You must increase the size and strength of the large muscle groups that compose the hips and thighs.

Hot Hips and Fabulous Thighs does both. Best of all, it does both simultaneously.

···8···

Realistic Goals

:

You've seen the before-and-after photographs in this book. You've examined the possibilities and you've made up your mind that you're going to get great results.

Before you go forward, however, it's a good idea to have some realistic goals for yourself.

••• WHAT TO EXPECT

In 1989 and 1990, 118 women took part in the research for this book. Before-and-after measurements for the 118 women show that, in six weeks, each lost an average of:

- 12 pounds of fat
- 1 ³/₄ inches off the hips
- 2 ¹/₂ inches off the upper thighs
- 2 inches off the middle thighs
- 2 ¹/₂ inches off the waist

These same women added an average of 3 pounds of figure-enhancing muscle to their lower bodies. The above averages provide realistic expectations for most women motivated to follow the week-by-week plan. Some women can expect less results and some can achieve greater results, even as much as doubling the average expectations.

For maximum benefits, follow the program exactly as it is presented. First, it's important that you accurately assess your body fat and body measurements.

29

••• BODY FAT PERCENTAGE

Since most of your fat is stored directly under the skin, measuring the thickness of skin and fat is a way to determine body fatness. Here's how to measure:

1. Stand with your weight mostly on your left leg. Locate the skinfold site on the front of your right thigh midway between your hip and knee joints.

2. Lean forward and grasp a vertical fold of skin between your thumb and first finger. The fold should not include any muscle, just skin and fat. Practice pinching and pulling the skin until no muscle is included.

3. Pick up a ruler in your other hand. Measure the thickness of the skinfold to the nearest 1/8 inch by measuring the distance between your thumb and finger. Occasionally the top of the skinfold is thicker than the distance between your thumb and finger. To avoid this, keep the top of the skinfold level with the top of your thumb. Don't press the ruler against the skinfold, as this will flatten it out and make it appear thicker than it really is.

4. Take two separate measures of skinfold thickness, releasing the skin between each measure. Add them together and divide by two to determine the average thickness.

5. Estimate your percent body fat from the chart below.

1/2 inch	=	8–13%
7/8 inch	=	13–18%
1 1/4 inches	=	18–23%
1 5/8 inches	=	23–28%
2 1/4 inches	=	28–33%
2 3/4 inches	=	33–38%
3 1/8 inches	=	38–43%

Ideally, your skinfold thickness on your thigh should be 7/8 inch or less. This means that your body fat level is below 18 percent, which is excellent. Within reason, the less fat you have under your skin and around your thighs, the better off you are physically. As your thigh skinfold gets smaller, your waist, thighs, hips, and overall body will automatically develop a tighter, more muscular appearance.

••• BODY MEASUREMENTS

It is important to take your before-and-after body measurements and enter them on the chart on pages 33 and 34.

1. Measure your height and weight.

2. Take relaxed circumference measurements at nine sites: both upper arms midway between your elbow and shoulder; chest at nipple level; waist at your naval; hips with heels together; both thighs just below your buttocks; and both thighs midway between your hip and knee joints. Apply the tape firmly but do not compress the skin. Do not take measurements over clothes and do not work out before measuring.

3. Determine total fat loss at the end of the program by multiplying percentage of body fat times body weight for the before-and-after tests. For example, if you weighed 140 pounds with 28 percent body fat at the start of the program, that's 39.2 pounds of fat. If you completed the program at 125 pounds and 18 percent body fat, that's 22.5 pounds of fat. The difference between 39.2 and 22.5 is 16.7 pounds of total fat loss.

4. Calculate the amount of muscle gained by subtracting the weight lost from the total fat lost. In the example above, where fat loss equaled 16.7 pounds and weight loss equaled 15 pounds, 1.7 pounds of muscle were gained.

••• BEFORE-AND-AFTER PHOTOGRAPHS

One of the most meaningful things you can do is to take before-and-after pictures of yourself in a tight bathing suit. You'll be able to see with your own eyes the positive results of this six-week plan.

Here are the guidelines to follow:

1. Have your photographer use a 35-millimeter camera, if possible, loaded with black-and-white print film. He should turn the camera sideways for a vertical format negative.

2. Wear a snug bathing suit (a solid color is best) and stand against an uncluttered, light background.

3. Have the photographer move away from you until he can see your entire body in the viewfinder. He should sit in a chair and hold the camera level with your navel, preferably mounting the camera at this level on a tripod.

4. Pose in three directions: front, side, and back, with your hands on top of your head in each shot and feet spaced apart evenly.

5. Repeat the photo session in six weeks, wearing the same bathing suit and assuming identical poses.

6. Instruct the photo processor to make your after prints exactly the same size as your before prints. *Important:* your height in all the before-and-after photos must be standardized for valid comparisons to be made and fat losses noted. This is done by comparison cropping at the processing lab.

••• TIGHT PANTS TEST

An interesting test that I highly recommend is done with a tight pair of pants. Before you begin the course, squeeze into your tightest pair of pants. You'll probably have to do so by lying on the bed and sucking in your stomach. Stand up in front of a full-length mirror and have a good look. Etch in your mind how the pants look and feel.

Take the pants off and set them aside in a safe place. At the end of each of the program's two-week phases, slip back into the pants for another fitting. If you're following the program strictly, the pants should get looser and looser.

••• THE BOTTOM LINE

Percent body fat, total fat lost, muscle gained, inches lost, and full-body photos can indeed be perplexing. In a nutshell, however, here is the bottom line:

- if you have more than 1 inch of fat (skinfold thickness) on the middle of your thigh,

or

- if your hip measurement is significantly larger than 36 inches,

then

you are a prime candidate for Hot Hips and Fabulous Thighs!

HOT HIPS AND FABULOUS THIGHS
BEFORE-AND-AFTER MEASUREMENTS

Name ———————————————— Age ——————————

Date ———————————————— Height ——————————

SKINFOLD

	Before	After	Difference
Right Front Thigh	———	———	———
Percentage	———	———	———
Fat Pounds	———	———	———

BODY WEIGHT

Before	After	Difference
———	———	———

TOTAL FAT LOSS ————————

MUSCLE GAINED ————————

CIRCUMFERENCE MEASUREMENTS
—————————— • • • ——————————

	Before	After	Inches Lost
Right Arm	_____	_____	_____
Left Arm	_____	_____	_____
Chest	_____	_____	_____
Waist at Navel	_____	_____	_____
Hips	_____	_____	_____
Right Thigh (high)	_____	_____	_____
Left Thigh (high)	_____	_____	_____
Right Thigh (middle)	_____	_____	_____
Left Thigh (middle)	_____	_____	_____

TOTAL INCHES LOST   _____

···**9**···
Eating
for Fat Loss

The average woman, as discussed in Chapter 4, gains 1.5 pounds of fat each year. Although this seems like a small amount, over ten years it adds up to 15 pounds. And 15 pounds of fat, combined with a loss of 5 pounds of supporting muscle, can make a big difference in the way she looks.

An essential part of the Hot Hips and Fabulous Thighs program is to get rid of your excessive fat. Doing this requires the right type of diet and the right type of exercise. Chapter 11 details proper exercise. This chapter covers proper diet.

··· COMPONENTS OF A SOUND DIET

The Hot Hips and Fabulous Thighs diet, like the other eating plans I've designed over the last 15 years, works because it adheres to well-established criteria. A sound diet:

- Protects your health by supplying you with all the well-balanced nutrients you need.
- Provides you with enough calories to exercise intensely—from 1,400 to 1,000 calories per day—but at the same time allows you to lose fat effectively.
- Offers ample variety so boredom won't drive you to give up on the diet.
- Consists of ordinary foods available in supermarkets at reasonable prices.
- Teaches you good eating habits so you can keep the lost fat off permanently.

••• DESCENDING CALORIES

At the heart of the eating plan is a descending-calorie diet. Women who weigh more than 120 pounds, start with 1,400 calories a day for Weeks 1 and 2. Women who weigh under 120 pounds, begin with 1,200 calories a day. During Weeks 3 and 4 the calories are reduced by 100, and again by another 100 calories during Weeks 5 and 6.

Many women actually get fatter because they eat too few calories. Eating too little can cause your body to panic and start preserving fat. This descending-calorie diet was specifically calculated to prevent fat storage from happening. Furthermore, the descending-calorie plan makes the diet particularly good to use in conjunction with the Hot Hips and Fabulous Thighs exercise routine.

••• WELL-BALANCED EATING

The Hot Hips and Fabulous Thighs diet is well balanced. Each day you'll be consuming several servings from the Basic Four food groups. The groups are based on an excellent program originally developed by the U.S. Department of Agriculture in the 1950s and improved since then. The four categories are as follows:

- *Meat Group:* meat, poultry, fish, eggs, and legumes such as dried beans, peas, lentils
- *Milk Group:* milk, yogurt, cheese
- *Fruits and Vegetables Group*
- *Breads and Cereals Group:* grains, cereals, rice, pasta

For six weeks, you are given menus designed to meet an approximate 2:2:4:4 ratio of Meat to Milk to Fruits and Vegetables to Breads and Cereals. A 2:2:4:4 ratio means that your daily caloric intake will be approximately 50 percent carbohydrates, 30 percent fats, and 20 percent proteins—a diet pattern good for life. Whether or not you are dieting, the basic proportioning of food groups in this plan is the key to eating nutritionally balanced meals.

The emphasis of the Basic Four is on what you should eat. Nutritionists also recognize a fifth food group—labeled "Other"— made up of foods to consume in small amounts. The Other category contains fats, sugars, and alcohol. Consuming these foods can provide you with ample calories but insufficient amounts of essential vitamins and minerals.

Fats, sugars, and alcohol are calorie-dense, providing more calories than nutrients. Fats (such as butter, margarine, oils, and salad dressings) are often referred to as concentrated calories because, gram for gram, they contain more than twice the calories of either proteins or carbohydrates. You should not cut fats from your diet altogether. Moderate amounts of fat provide a feeling of satisfaction, or satiety, which is very important over the long haul because it keeps you on the diet. Part of your fat allotment each day is built into foods from the Basic Four food groups. Milk, meat, and most breads contain fat. In examining the menus, notice that you'll be adding only small quantities of fat to that which you'll be getting from the Basic Four.

•• SMALL MEALS PLUS SNACKS

Research shows that many small meals a day are more effective for losing fat than several larger meals. In other words, you should eat something every three to five hours that you are awake. This concept is used in the Hot Hips and Fabulous Thighs eating plan.

The menus presented in later chapters are composed of the usual meals: breakfast, lunch, and dinner. In addition, there are between-meal snacks that are nutritionally important.

Your appetite will be appeased on this diet and you'll rarely suffer from an empty feeling in your stomach. It is important, however, that you follow the meal and snack suggestions exactly as presented for best results.

Besides the food you eat, another salient nutritional component in losing fat is water. You'll find out why in the next chapter.

···**10**···

Water
Your Fat Away

Reading this chapter can make you thirsty. And it should. Because water is your body's most precious nutrient. It is not only essential for life, but also necessary for efficient fat loss.

If you don't drink enough water, your body's reaction is to retain what water is does have. This, in turn, hampers kidney function, and waste products accumulate. The liver is then called upon to help flush out the impurities. As a result, one of the liver's major functions—metabolizing stored body fat into usable energy—is minimized. Thus, a fat buildup occurs, water is retained, and body weight soars.

To combat this fat buildup and to facilitate the loss of fat, you must drink more water than you probably believe you need.

··● MORE THAN EIGHT GLASSES

The standard recommendation for water is to drink eight 8-ounce glasses a day. During periods of fat loss and intense exercise that's not nearly enough. That's why I recommend that dieters on the Hot Hips and Fabulous Thighs program consume from 16 to 26 glasses (1 to 1 5/8 gallons) of water a day. The specifics of how to do this will be explained in Chapter 15.

It may help you to purchase a plastic water bottle, the kind with a straw, readily available in supermarkets, service stations, and convenience stores. With such a bottle, you can carry water with you throughout the day for continuous drinking.

To further improve your fat-loss results the water you drink should be ice cold. A gallon of cold water (40 degrees Fahrenheit) requires approximately 200 calories of heat energy to warm it to core body temperature (98.6 degrees Fahrenheit). The water goes in cold and comes out warm.

Water is very important to an exercise program because it gives muscles their natural ability to contract. From 70 to 75 percent of your muscle mass is composed of water. That's one reason you get thirsty when you exercise.

Water also helps to prevent the sagging skin that usually follows fat loss. Shrinking cells are buoyed by this fluid, which plumps the skin and leaves it clear, healthy, and resilient.

•• THIRST

You should drink plenty of water even if you're not thirsty. Responding to thirst will prevent only severe dehydration. It will not prompt you to drink the water you need to function at your peak.

Inadequate water intake causes the body to perceive a threat to survival, and thus it begins to hold on to every drop. Water is then stored outside the cells, showing up as swollen feet, legs or hands—what we commonly refer to as water retention.

The best way to overcome water retention is to give your body the water it needs. Only then will stored water be released.

If you have a persistent problem with water retention, even after drinking at least sixteen glasses a day, excess sodium is probably to blame. The more sodium you ingest, the more water your system retains to dilute it.

One source of sodium not to be overlooked is your favorite diet soda. Although free from sugar, the sodium in diet drinks may cause water retention. Carefully check the labels to make certain these drinks contain little or no sodium.

•• FEELING FULL

Overeating can also be averted through water intake. Water can keep your stomach feeling full and satisfied between meals, thus preventing it from signaling your brain that you are hungry. When water is consumed in conjunction with foods high in fiber, this satisfied feeling increases because the fiber in these foods actually absorbs the water and swells in size.

•• CONSTIPATION CURE

Another desirable side effect of increased water intake is its effect on constipation. An article in a national magazine suggested recently that "nearly 90 percent of overweight women suffer from constipation."

Restricting your water intake makes you constipated. When deprived of water, your system pulls it from your lower intestines and bowel—thus creating hard, dry stools.

Water helps rid the body of waste, which is even more critical during periods of fat reduction since metabolized fat must be shed.

•• RUNNING TO THE BATHROOM

You're probably wondering: if you drink from 16 to 26 glasses of water a day, won't you be running back and forth to the bathroom all day long?

Initially, for two weeks or so, your bladder will be hypersensitive to the increased amount of fluid. And yes, you will have to urinate frequently. Soon your bladder will calm down and you will urinate less frequently but in larger amounts.

•• WATER VERSUS OTHER BEVERAGES

There is a difference between water and other beverages that contain water. Biochemically, water is water. Obviously you can get it consuming such beverages as soft drinks, tea, coffee, beer, and fruit juices. While such drinks contain water, they also have substances that contradict some of the positive effects of the added water.

Soft drinks, coffee, and tea can contain caffeine, which stimulates the adrenal glands and acts as a diuretic. Some beverages are loaded with sugar and alcohol calories. In addition, too many flavored drinks can decrease your taste for water.

*"***M****y fat loss began to accelerate when I started drinking over a gallon of water a day. I never believed you could water your body and grow thin, but you can. "*

SUZANNE FOREMAN
— • • —

age: 26
height: 5'9"

LOST 13½ pounds of fat, **RESHAPED** her body by adding 3 pounds of muscle, and **TRIMMED** 2 inches off her waist, 2½ inches off her hips, and 3 inches off her upper thighs in six weeks.

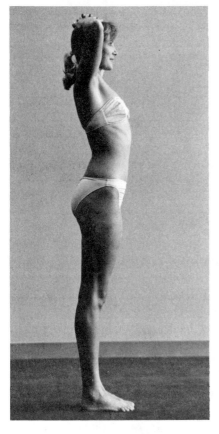 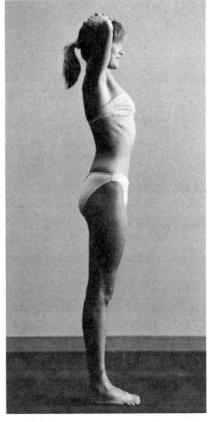

Before   **After**

The way to interpret all of this is that your recommended daily water intake means just that—water!

••• TAP WATER OR BOTTLED WATER

In general, the United States has one of the safest water supplies in the world. Chances are high that your community's tap water is fine for drinking.

Furthermore, research shows that bottled water is not always higher-quality water than tap water. The decision to drink bottled water or not is usually one of taste.

If you dislike the taste of your tap water, then drink your favorite bottled water. If you have no problems with your city's water supply, then save some money and consume it.

••• THREE IMPORTANT STEPS

Effective and efficient fat loss requires that you:

1. Drink water
2. Drink more water
3. Drink even more water

Remember—water will help to wash your fat away.

••• A FINAL NOTE

Although it is doubtful that you could ever drink too much water (you'd throw it up or simply urinate more), a few ailments can be negatively affected by large amounts of fluid. Before consuming the recommended 16 to 26 glasses of water a day on this program, play it safe and check with your personal physician.

···11···
Exercising for Fat Loss

•
•
•

Muscle-building activity is the best type of exercise for fat loss.

Why? Because more than any other component of your body that you have control over, your muscles require calories:

- Calories to keep warm
- Calories to regulate
- Calories to move
- Calories to recover
- Calories to grow

Add a pound of muscle to your body and you automatically require an extra 75 calories per day just to keep it alive. Add four pounds of muscle to your body—and it's quite possible to do so in only six weeks—and your resting metabolic rate increases by 300 calories per day.

Muscle is 37.5 times more metabolically active than the same amount of fat. A pound of fat on your body needs only 2 calories a day to keep it functioning.

Your muscles produce energy and create power, using calories to do so.

The best exercises for building your muscles are also the best exercises for losing fat.

••• FAT-BURNING EXERCISE

Your body produces energy primarily from carbohydrates (stored in the muscles as glycogen) and fats (circulating in your blood as free fatty acids). When you're at rest, your body uses approximately 60 percent free fatty acids and 40 percent carbohydrates to keep you functioning. When you work moderately, your body uses about a 50/50 ratio of fats to carbohydrates. As the workout becomes more challenging, or higher in intensity, it uses more and more carbohydrates to supply energy needs.

No matter which system your body is using, it burns calories when it produces energy. This can come from foods eaten, carbohydrates stored in the liver, and from fat cells. Fat cells produce free fatty acids and a molecule that forms proteins that can eventually be converted to replace carbohydrate stores. That's why during muscle-building exercise, even though the body relies largely on carbohydrates for energy production, you'll still lose fat. Those carbohydrates expended during exercise are replaced by foods eaten, and fat stores are mobilized to supply energy needs created by the deficit that occurs from your exercise performance and dietary restrictions.

••• MUSCLE-BUILDING EXERCISE

For an exercise to provide maximum muscle-building effects it must be intense, progressive, and long-range. Let's examine each characteristic.

Intense: High-intensity exercise is neither easy nor fun. It is demanding. These demands cause labored breathing, increased pulse, elevated blood pressure, heightened metabolic rate, and pronounced muscle burn. Such an intense effort should lead to momentary muscular fatigue in a major muscle in approximately 60 to 180 seconds.

Progressive: There must be a relatively easy way to progress by making the exercise harder. Such progression is accomplished by adding a small amount of weight to the exercise implement. The implement is usually a dumbbell, barbell, exercise machine, or your own body weight. Alternatives to adding weight are to increase the repetitions or elapsed time, and to slow down the speed of movement.

Long-Range: A deep knee bend or squat is a long-range exercise. As you bend your knees and hips, your buttocks go low and almost touch your heels. You then smoothly straighten your knees

and hips and return to the standing position. Lowering your buttocks one-fourth or one-half of the way down is an example of a
short-range exercise. It should be obvious that long-range exercises are harder, more thorough, and more productive on the involved muscles than short-range or partial-range exercises.

Many traditional-type exercises for women are not intense
enough, progressive enough, or long-range enough to produce
much in the way of muscle building. Aerobic dancing, floor exercises, jogging, cycling, swimming, and stair climbing all fall into
this category.

The Hot Hips and Fabulous Thighs program, on the other hand,
is intense, progressive, and long-range. It does stimulate your muscles to grow.

Remember, larger muscles are firmer and more shapely . . .
and more fat burning.

•• ONLY THREE DAYS A WEEK

Stimulated muscles need time to get larger and stronger. It usually
takes a minimum of 48 hours for your body to recover fully from a
high-intensity workout. That's why the Hot Hips and Fabulous
Thighs exercise routine is only practiced three times a week:

Monday-Wednesday-Friday
or
Tuesday-Thursday-Saturday

Don't make the mistake of trying to do the routine more often.
It will not speed results. It could, in fact, actually hinder progress
by using up your recovery ability, as too much exercise can leave
your body in a state of overtraining. If this is the case, you will
soon lose your enthusiasm and break your diet.

••• NO SPECIAL EQUIPMENT

For those of you who want to do the exercise program at home, you
can do so without any special equipment. All it takes is a smooth
wall, a clock with a second hand that is large enough to see clearly
from 15 feet away, and a cushioned mat or carpet to lie on for floor
exercises. See Chapter 23 for all the details.

It is also possible to team up with a group of women and do the exercises together in a large room, or even perhaps at your local fitness center. Several fitness centers in Dallas offered Hot Hips and Fabulous Thighs under supervised conditions and had excellent results.

If you're a member of a fitness center, you may want to do your muscle-building exercise on their Nautilus equipment. If so, Chapter 24 illustrates the exercises to perform.

Whether you exercise at home or in a fitness center, you can still expect to add several pounds of body-shaping muscle to your hips and thighs—*if you perform the exercises properly*. Proper performance of each exercise is crucial for maximum results. The key concept in proper performance is moving *super slow,* which is the subject of the next chapter.

···12···
Slow Down, You Move Too Fast

:

Aerobic dancing. Jazzercise. Bench stepping. Stair climbing. Calisthenics. Floor exercises. Heavy hands. Free-weight lifting. Nautilus training.

Millions of women are involved weekly in performing the above exercises in a rapid and jerky manner. They would get much better results if they slowed their speed of movement. A slow speed of movement is more productive and safer.

··• MORE PRODUCTIVE

When you move slowly during an exercise, you significantly reduce the momentum that normally occurs. As a result, you activate parts of the muscle that are not usually brought into action. Activating these dormant muscle cells is what stimulates them to get larger, stronger, firmer, and more shapely. This is especially important in training the hips and thighs.

··• SAFER

Injuries are usually caused by excessive force. Yanking, jerking, and moving suddenly while exercising is not safe. When a force exceeds the structural integrity of your body, something usually breaks.

It is far better to lift and lower your body weight, or an exercise machine, in a smooth and controlled fashion. Thus, the force on the muscle remains steady and much safer than the traditional faster, jerky styles of exercising.

••• IDEAL SPEED OF MOVEMENT

Most advanced exercisers think of momentum in terms of highly explosive movement. In reality, it's much more subtle than that. Momentum is involved in even moderately paced movement.

Researchers Ken and Brenda Hutchins, with whom I've worked frequently on my diet and exercise programs, found that the speed of movement producing the least momentum, and consequently the best results, was approximately 10 seconds to lift the resistance and 5 seconds to lower the same resistance. The resistance could be in the form of a barbell, dumbbell, weight machine, or your own body weight.

Additional research with body weight and floor exercises proved that holding your body stationary with sustained muscular contraction in certain positions improved the intensity of the exercise. Particular emphasis in each exercise is applied to pausing and squeezing at the fully contracted position.

••• SUPER SLOW

This smooth, deliberate way of exercising is called *super slow,* and it was principally developed by Ken Hutchins. The specifics of each of the recommended hip and thigh exercises will be described in Chapters 23 and 24.

Move slower, never faster, if in doubt about your speed. This is one of the basic principles of efficient muscle building. Yet it is often one of the first violated by most trainees because it is easier to move fast and jerky than it is to move slowly and smoothly. Superslow repetitions soon become a painful, fatiguing experience.

While you are exercising, remember that:

- *Slow, intense exercise is the best way to build your muscles.*
- *Bigger, stronger muscles burn more fat around your hips and thighs.*

Decide now that you want to get maximum results from your exercise. Slow down!

···13···

Synergy:
One Plus One = Five

⋮

The Hot Hips and Fabulous Thighs program produces synergy. Synergy is the simultaneous occurrence of separate factors that together create greater total effect than the sum of their individual actions.

Enthusiastic involvement in this program evokes at least five benefits: guaranteed fat loss, increased metabolic rate, improved body shape, enhanced self-esteem, and reformed diet and exercise habits.

••• GUARANTEED FAT LOSS

Guaranteed fat loss means that weight lost from the Hot Hips and Fabulous Thighs program is entirely from stored fat. Most other plans produce weight losses not solely from fat but from significant reductions in fluids and tissues. Losing fluids from muscles, blood, and organs is dangerous. The best way to ensure that weight loss is completely from stored fat is to stimulate your muscles to grow, using fat as a source of energy for growth.

How does strengthening muscle guarantee your weight loss will be from fat?

An animal study published by Dr. Alfred Goldberg and colleagues in a 1975 issue of *Medicine and Science in Sports* details the process. Dr. Goldberg found that if muscle is stimulated to grow through exercise, it will grow in defiance of tremendous adversity—even at the expense of the remainder of the organism.

A fundamental trait of animal life is locomotion, which depends on muscular size and strength. Survival resources are allocated to the muscles first. This priority allocation depends, however, on muscle stimulation. Without that stimulation, resources are stored, passed out, or put to other uses.

The same physiology is in operation within the human body. When you embark on a low-calorie diet, your body perceives that something is wrong. It starts preserving fat as a survival mechanism. This is why so many women can't lose fat even though they're barely eating. To prevent this from occurring, you must overrule your survival mechanism by stimulating muscle growth. Your muscles will then pull calories from your fat cells and your weight loss will be entirely from fat.

••• INCREASED METABOLIC RATE

Both muscle and fat require calories for vital functioning. Muscle is very active metabolically. Fat is just the opposite—almost dormant. Recall that a gain of one pound of muscle raises your metabolic rate by approximately 75 calories per day. Muscle burns 37.5 times more calories per day than an equal amount of fat, which burns only 2 calories a day per pound.

As your muscles grow larger—and they will from the prescribed exercise—your metabolic rate will increase. Your new body, with extra muscle, will burn more calories.

Your maintenance plan for permanent weight control can include many of your favorite foods and drinks. With additional muscles demanding extra calories daily just for maintenance, you can eat normally without regaining your lost fat.

••• IMPROVED BODY SHAPE

Probably the most gratifying result of this program is improved body shape. Body shape is primarily dependent on your muscle-to-fat ratio, as was discussed in Chapter 4. Most women over twenty have too little muscle and too much fat. Gaining muscle and losing fat dramatically improves the appearance of your figure, especially your hips and thighs. The confidence you have in your body impacts you physically, mentally, and socially. When you reshape your figure, you'll look better, feel better, and perform better.

••• ENHANCED SELF-ESTEEM

When you lose fat, build muscle, and slim and firm your hips and thighs, you also significantly enhance your self-esteem. Because you have accomplished something meaningful, and because doing so involved hard work, you have greater belief in yourself. This belief turns into what I call healthy pride.

"The reason I did this program," said Cherry Reck of Orlando, who dropped several dress sizes, "was for myself. I have a full-length mirror in my bedroom and I didn't like what I saw. Now, I not only like what I see, but the compliments are almost unbelievable. My self-esteem is soaring."

••• REFORMED DIETING AND EXERCISING HABITS

The process of reaching your fat-loss and body-shaping goals gradually reforms your dieting and exercising habits. The same mechanics that you employ during the six-week program can be used throughout your life.

The basics of proper eating and proper exercising are not concepts that are tried and discarded. These fundamentals are designed to become vital habits that lead to long-lasting results.

You can expect your life to change, and it will for the better—thanks to *SYNERGY*—in only six weeks!

···14···

More Visual Proof

:

Surveys show that nine out of ten women are reluctant to wear a bathing suit; one out of three shuns bright colors; more than half avoid wearing slacks and shorts.

The reason?

Their hips and thighs are too big. These body parts are laden with fat and lacking in muscle tone.

Still, most of these women have dreams: dreams of firm, shapely buttocks, dreams of long, lean thighs. In their minds they know it's unrealistic to imitate a size-7 model, but in their dreams they'd like to look like she does.

If your dreams are realistic, and if you work hard enough—in an intelligent manner—your goals can become realities.

Here are six women who went through the six-week program. Each one had a dream, a dream of Hot Hips and Fabulous Thighs. Each one took major steps toward her goals.

*"**A** little bit of muscle goes a long way, especially if it's in the right places. The program has really firmed and tightened my thighs."*

MARY HAGER
•••

age: 30
height: 5'4"

LOST 12 1/4 pounds of fat, **RESHAPED** her body by adding 1 3/4 pounds of muscle, and **TRIMMED** 3 1/8 inches off her waist, 2 1/8 inches off her hips, and 3 1/2 inches off her upper thighs in six weeks.

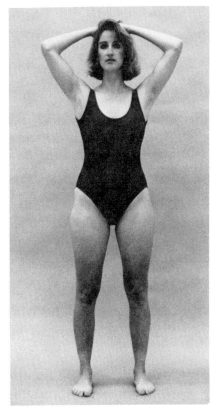 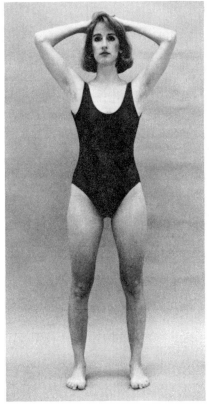

Before   **After**

"I feel much stronger in my lower body. My confidence has improved, too."

DEE DEE THOMASSON
•••

age: 29
height: 5'5"

LOST 10 1/2 pounds of fat, **RESHAPED** her body by adding 1 1/2 pounds of muscle, and **TRIMMED** 4 3/8 inches off her waist, 1 5/8 inches off her hips, and 3 3/4 inches off her upper thighs in six weeks.

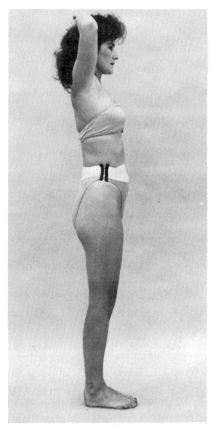 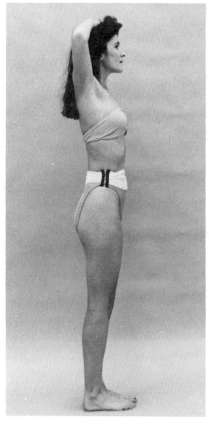

Before   **After**

"All my clothes fit so much better. My friends have noticed the difference in my appearance."

VICKI McCORMACK
—•••—

age: 32
height: 5'3"

LOST 9 1/2 pounds of fat, **RESHAPED** her body by adding 1 1/2 pounds of muscle, and **TRIMMED** 1 3/4 inches off her waist, 2 1/4 inches off her hips, and 3 7/8 inches off her upper thighs in six weeks.

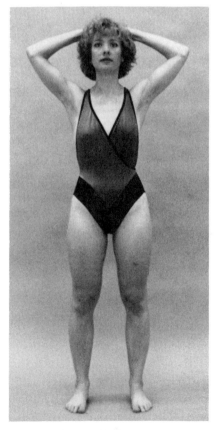 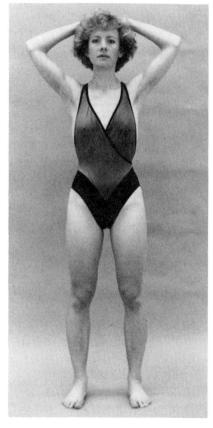

Before   **After**

"I've had those ripples on my back thighs for years. In six weeks they've gone."

ELLEN COLLELUORI
— •●• —

age: 30
height: 5'4"

LOST 11 ½ pounds of fat, **RESHAPED** her body by adding ½ pound of muscle, and **TRIMMED** 1 ³/₈ inches off her waist, 2 ⁵/₈ inches off her hips, and 4 ½ inches off her upper thighs in six weeks.

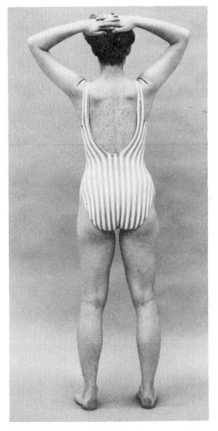 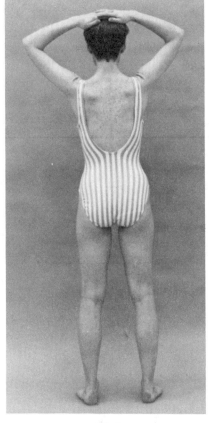

Before   **After**

"The Hot Hips and Fabulous Thighs program has made a big difference in the way I look, feel, and act. Even my posture has improved."

KAREN COOPER
•••

age: 30
height: 5'7 ½"

LOST 17 ½ pounds of fat, **RESHAPED** her body by adding 4 pounds of muscle, and **TRIMMED** 2 ½ inches off her waist, 2 ¾ inches off her hips, and 4 inches off her upper thighs in six weeks.

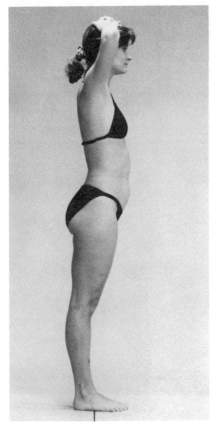
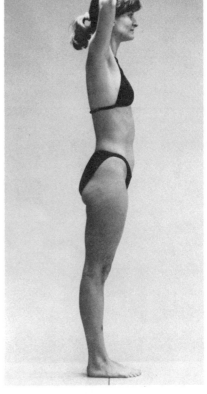

Before   **After**

"I used to feel fat and flabby. Not anymore! I reshaped my body and my confidence."

JULIA KLUG
—————•●•—————

age: 31
height: 5′4½″

LOST 11 pounds of fat, **RESHAPED** her body by adding 1¼ pounds of muscle, and **TRIMMED** 2⅜ inches off her waist, 1¾ inches off her hips, and 2 inches off her upper thighs in six weeks.

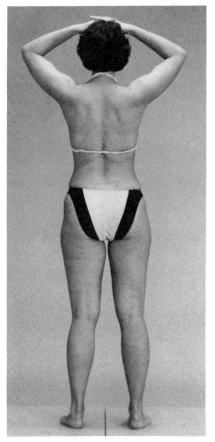 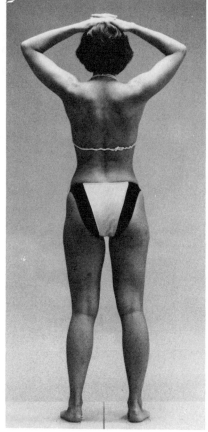

Before   **After**

···15···
Before Starting the Program

:

There are a number of important steps to take before starting the Hot Hips and Fabulous Thighs plan. Devoting the necessary attention to each step will make it easier for you to reach your goal.

••• GET YOUR DOCTOR'S PERMISSION

Before you begin this program, be sure your doctor knows you plan to modify both your eating and exercising habits. Show him this book so he's aware of what's involved. He'll likely recommend a thorough physical examination if he hasn't given you one in the last year.

There are a few people who should not try the program: children and teenagers; women with certain types of heart, liver, or kidney disease; diabetics; and those suffering from some types of arthritis. This should not be taken as an all-inclusive list. Some women should follow the course only with their physician's specific guidance and recommendations. Consult your doctor beforehand to play it safe.

••• DO YOUR "BEFORE" MEASUREMENTS AND PHOTOGRAPHS

Don't procrastinate on taking your measurements and photographs. Without accurate assessments, you'll be traveling a difficult road without a good support system. Get out your bathing suit, tape measure, and camera and do it now.

Every dieter who has neglected this procedure has regretted it later when, after reshaping her body, she had no concrete documentation of her efforts.

•• BUY FOOD MEASURING SPOONS, CUPS, AND A SMALL SCALE

Most people overestimate one-half cup of orange juice, one tablespoon of raisins, or one ounce of mozzarella cheese. Such practices lead to sloppy recipe preparation, inaccurate calorie counting, and inefficient fat loss. It is important to become familiar with and correctly use measuring spoons, cups, and food scales.

All of these items can be purchased inexpensively at your local department store or supermarket. With food scales, however, you'd be well advised to spend more money to purchase a battery-operated, digital scale instead of the less expensive, spring-loaded type. The accuracy of the digital scale could lead to extra inches off your hips and thighs.

•• TAKE A VITAMIN-MINERAL TABLET EACH DAY

Although the Hot Hips and Fabulous Thighs diet is well balanced, you should take *one* multiple vitamin-with-minerals tablet each morning. Be certain no nutrient listed on the label exceeds 100 percent of the U.S. Recommended Daily Allowances. High-potency supplements are a waste of money.

•• EXAMINE THE MENUS, RECIPES, AND SHOPPING LISTS

Glance through the menus, recipes, and shopping lists (Chapters 16 through 20) for an overview of what you'll be eating during the next six weeks. Your results will be more effective if you plan ahead.

•• KEEP FOOD SUBSTITUTIONS TO A MINIMUM

I recommend that you follow the menus and recipes exactly as indicated. The women who obtain the best results almost never vary from the listed foods. I know there are times when some women must make substitutions for certain foods. For example, those who are allergic to milk may substitute one ounce of cheese or one cup of low-fat yogurt for one cup of milk in any menu. Those who are vegetarians may exchange one egg or a cup of cooked dried beans or peas for one meat serving.

••• HAVE A FRIEND GO THROUGH THE PROGRAM WITH YOU

You'll probably get better fat-loss and muscle-building results if you go through the program with a friend. Both you and your friend should need about the same degree of fat loss. You should both be serious about making a six-week commitment. That commitment means you'll be exercising together three times a week, talking often on the phone, shopping together, monitoring each other's water intake, and sharing problems.

••• DRINK 16 TO 26 GLASSES OF COLD WATER EACH DAY

Do not underestimate the importance of drinking plenty of cold water. Invariably, the women who lose the most fat in six weeks have the highest daily water intakes.

You should begin your water drinking by consuming 16 glasses, or 1 gallon, a day for the first week. You then add 2 daily glasses a week until the end of the program, as indicated below:

**NUMBER OF EIGHT-OUNCE GLASSES
OF WATER PER DAY**

- Week 1 = 16
- Week 2 = 18
- Week 3 = 20

- Week 4 = 22
- Week 5 = 24
- Week 6 = 26

During Week 6 you're consuming 26 glasses, 208 ounces, or 1 5/8 gallons of water a day. You may believe that it's impossible to drink 26 glasses of water. It probably would be if you tried to force it down at one time. The secret is to spread it out and drink 75 to 80 percent of the water before 5:00 p.m.

Here's a weekly water-drinking schedule that many women find helpful:

WATER-DRINKING SCHEDULE
—•••—
NUMBER OF SIXTEEN-OUNCE BOTTLES PER DAY

Time	Wk1	Wk2	Wk3	Wk4	Wk5	Wk6
7:00 a.m.						
	3	4	4	4	5	5
12:00 Noon						
	3	3	4	4	4	5
5:00 p.m.						
	2	2	2	3	3	3
11:00 p.m.						
TOTAL: 16-ounce Bottles per day	8	9	10	11	12	13

Note: Drink 75–80 percent of water between 7:00 a.m. and 5:00 p.m.

A 16-ounce plastic bottle with a straw makes the procedure easier to follow. Most women find they can consume more fluid with a straw than they can by drinking from a glass. A great way to keep up with your water drinking is to place rubber bands around the middle of the bottle equal to the number of bottles of water you are supposed to drink. Each time you finish 16 ounces, take off a rubber band.

••• AVOID INTENSE ACTIVITY ON YOUR NON-EXERCISE DAYS

Too much activity can be more harmful to your body than too little activity, especially when you're following a low-calorie diet. If you exercise intensely more than three times per week, your system soon reaches a state of overtraining. Fat losses and strength gains slow rather than accelerate. You eventually get the blahs, have little enthusiasm, and break your diet. At this point you are close to "burning the candle at both ends, and trying to light it in the middle too."

During your participation in the Hot Hips and Fabulous Thighs program, it is to your advantage to keep your outside endeavors to a minimum. Naturally, you can continue with your normal work and household responsibilities. Simply avoid vigorous activities such as running, skiing, racquetball, and aerobic dancing. Light recreation is fine. Once you reach your fat-loss goals, you can get involved in strenuous sports and fitness activities if you wish.

••• BE PATIENT

You are now well-prepared to begin the program. The next six weeks will make a difference in your life.

Be patient. You can achieve your goals.

···16···
Hip and Thigh Diet: Weeks 1 and 2

The calories you consume each day will gradually descend from 1,400 for Weeks 1 and 2, to 1,300 for Weeks 3 and 4, to 1,200 for Weeks 5 and 6. Such a descending-calorie eating plan is the most productive way to lose fat from your body.

Each day you'll be allowed only limited choices of foods for breakfast and lunch. I've found that most dieters can consume the same basic breakfast and the same basic lunch for months with little or no modification. During your evening meal, however, you'll be treated with ample variety, which will make your daily eating interesting and enjoyable.

Included in the evening menu entrees are three meals centered around frozen dinners. This convenience factor will minimize those hectic schedule problems that most participants face. Each dinner selection fits the requirements of the Hot Hips and Fabulous Thighs program, as well as being within the suggested nutrition guidelines of the Surgeon General. Furthermore, on the Hot Hips and Fabulous Thighs program, you'll always have a mid-afternoon and late-night snack.

Begin Week 1 on Monday and continue through Sunday. Week 2 is an exact repeat of Week 1. Calories for each food are noted in parentheses. An asterisk (*) preceding a listing indicates that a recipe for that dish may be found in Chapter 19. A shopping list is provided in Chapter 20 to assist you.

Note: If you weigh 120 pounds or under, you'll need to adapt the diet slightly by applying the guidelines in Chapter 21.

••• A SIMPLE PLAN

The basic plan calls for six eating episodes per day. The system works as follows:

- *Breakfast:* There are two breakfast choices during the first two weeks, then four choices during the middle two weeks, and six choices during Weeks 5 and 6. All choices are 255 calories.

- *Mid-morning snack:* The mid-morning snack changes every two weeks. During Weeks 1–4 the calorie total is 102, and 45 calories the last two weeks.

- *Lunch:* Two basic lunch choices during Weeks 1 and 2, then four choices during the middle two weeks, and five choices during Weeks 5 and 6. All choices are 352 calories.

- *Afternoon snack:* There are two choices each week for an afternoon snack: an apple or pineapple and raisins. During the first two weeks enjoy an apple that is 3 inches in diameter or 2 slices of pineapple and 1 tablespoon of raisins. Each totals 100 calories. During Weeks 3–6, switch to ½ cup unsweetened applesauce or half of a fresh or canned pear.

- *Dinner:* For each night of the week there is a different dinner of approximately 400 calories. These should follow the same rotation each seven days. In some cases the main dinner course will be a commercially available frozen entree. Other dinners contain recipes for the main and side dishes. An optional dinner may be substituted during the third and fifth weeks.

- *Evening snack:* The evening snack changes every two weeks.

Follow the eating plan carefully to make sure you consume the appropriate foods at the recommended intervals.

MENUS FOR WEEKS 1 AND 2
————————— • • • —————————

MONDAY, Total calories, including snacks: 1,398

- **Breakfast:**   255 calories
  - **Basic Breakfast One**
    Cereal choices (1-ounce serving, 110 calories):
    Nabisco Shredded Wheat
    Kellogg's Frosted Mini-Wheats
    Kellogg's NutriGrain Wheat or Corn
    Post Grape Nuts
    Ralston Purina Almond Delight
    ³/₄ cup cooked oatmeal, sprinkled with cinnamon and
    low-calorie sweetener

    Plus
    ¹/₂ cup skim milk (45)
    1 slice reduced-calorie bread, toasted (40)
    ¹/₂ tablespoon low-calorie margarine (25)
    6 ounces low-calorie cranberry juice (35)
    or
    6 ounces vegetable juice cocktail (35)

  OR

  - **Basic Breakfast Two**
    8 ounces fruited, non-fat yogurt (any flavor), sweetened
    with aspartame (100)
    1 Nature Valley regular granola bar (Almond, Cinnamon,
    or Oats 'n Honey) (120)
    6 ounces low-calorie cranberry juice (35)
    or
    6 ounces vegetable juice cocktail (35)

- **Mid-morning Snack:**   102 calories
  - **Mid-morning Snack One**
  * 2 tablespoons Home Granola, Recipe #1 (50)
    2 tablespoons raisins (52)

  OR

  - **Mid-morning Snack Two**
  * Banana Snack Cake, Recipe #2 (85)
    1 teaspoon low-calorie margarine (17)

- **Lunch:**   352 calories
  - **Basic Lunch One**
  - Pasta-Stuffed Tomato, Recipe #3 (204)
    1/2 cup fruited, non-fat yogurt (any flavor), sweetened
    with aspartame (50)
    1/2 medium banana (8 3/4 inches long) (50)
    4 saltines (48)
    Noncaloric beverage

  OR

  - **Basic Lunch Two**
  - Chicken or Tuna or Turkey Salad Sandwich, Recipe #4
    (212)
    1/2 medium banana (8 3/4 inches long) (50)
    1 cup skim milk (90)

- **Mid-afternoon Fruit Snack:**   100 calories
  - **Fruit Snack One**
    1 medium apple (3-inch diameter) (100)
  OR

  - **Fruit Snack Two**
    1 tablespoon raisins (26)
    2 slices pineapple, juice-packed (70)

- **Dinner:**   394 calories
  Stouffer's Right Course Shrimp Primavera (240)
  Salad:
    Lettuce leaf (2)
    2 slices tomato (14)
    2 rings green pepper, 3-inch × 1/4-inch thick (4)
    1/2 cup cucumber, pared and diced (10)
    2 radishes, sliced (3)
  Creamy Italian Dressing:
    2 tablespoons non-fat yogurt (13)
    1 tablespoon diet Italian dressing (6)
  Garlic Bread:
    1 slice reduced-calorie bread (40)
    1 teaspoon low-calorie margarine (17)
    Sprinkling of powdered garlic or garlic salt
  1/4 cup applesauce, unsweetened (25), stir in
  1/3 cup strawberries, sliced (17)
  Noncaloric beverage

- **Evening Snack:** 195 calories
  - **Evening Snack One**
  - Tortilla Chips, Recipe #5 (use 2 1/2 corn tortillas) (175)
    1/4 cup salsa (20)
    Noncaloric beverage

OR

  - **Evening Snack Two**
    1 3/4 graham crackers (7 sections) (105)
    1 cup skim milk (90)

TUESDAY, Total calories, including snacks: 1,407

- **Breakfast:** 255 calories
  - Basic Breakfast One
    or
  - Basic Breakfast Two

- **Mid-morning Snack:** 102 calories
  - Mid-morning Snack One
    or
  - Mid-morning Snack Two

- **Lunch:** 352 calories
  - Basic Lunch One
    or
  - Basic Lunch Two

- **Mid-afternoon Fruit Snack:** 100 calories
  - Fruit Snack One
    or
  - Fruit Snack Two

- **Dinner:** 403 calories
  - Chicken Fajitas, Recipe #6 (328)
    1/2 cup canned peaches, juice-packed (50)
    1/2 cup strawberries, sliced (25)
    Noncaloric beverage

- **Evening Snack:**   195 calories
  - Evening Snack One
    or
  - Evening Snack Two

WEDNESDAY, Total calories, including snacks: 1,405

- **Breakfast:**   255 calories
  - Basic Breakfast One
    or
  - Basic Breakfast Two

- **Mid-morning Snack:**   102 calories

  - Mid-morning Snack One
    or
  - Mid-morning Snack Two

- **Lunch:**   352 calories
  - Basic Lunch One
    or
  - Basic Lunch Two

- **Mid-afternoon Fruit Snack:**   100 calories
  - Fruit Snack One
    or
  - Fruit Snack Two

- **Dinner:**   401 calories
  Le Menu, 3-Cheese Stuffed Shells (280)
  Salad:
  1 slice pineapple, juice-packed, chopped (35)
  1 tablespoon raisins (26)
  1 teaspoon low-calorie mayonnaise (13)
  1 lettuce leaf (2)
  ¾ graham cracker, 3 sections (45)
  Noncaloric beverage

- **Evening Snack:**   195 calories
  - Evening Snack One
    or
  - Evening Snack Two

THURSDAY, Total calories, including snacks: 1,394

- **Breakfast:** 255 calories
  - Basic Breakfast One
    or
  - Basic Breakfast Two

- **Mid-morning Snack:** 102 calories
  - Mid-morning Snack One
    or
  - Mid-morning Snack Two

- **Lunch:** 352 calories
  - Basic Lunch One
    or
  - Basic Lunch Two

- **Mid-afternoon Fruit Snack:** 100 calories
  - Fruit Snack One
    or
  - Fruit Snack Two

- **Dinner:** 390 calories
  - Krab-Stuffed Potato, Recipe #7 (218)
    1 cup chopped broccoli, steamed (40)
    1 slice reduced-calorie bread (40)
    1 teaspoon low-calorie margarine (17)
    ½ canned peach, juice-packed (50)
  - with 1 tablespoon Home Granola, Recipe #1 (25)
    Noncaloric beverage

- **Evening Snack:** 195 calories
  - Evening Snack One
    or
  - Evening Snack Two

FRIDAY, Total calories, including snacks: 1,404
- **Breakfast:** 255 calories

  - Basic Breakfast One
    or
  - Basic Breakfast Two

- **Mid-morning Snack:** 102 calories
  - Mid-morning Snack One
    or
  - Mid-morning Snack Two

- **Lunch:** 352 calories
  - Basic Lunch One
    or
  - Basic Lunch Two

- **Mid-afternoon Fruit Snack:** 100 calories
  - Fruit Snack One
    or
  - Fruit Snack Two

- **Dinner:** 400 calories
  Weight Watchers Deluxe Combination Pizza (320)
  Salad:
      1 cup lettuce, chopped (9)
      1 slice tomato (7)
      1 tablespoon diet Italian dressing (6)
      Sprinkle dried basil
      Sprinkle 1 teaspoon Parmesan cheese (8)
  $1/2$ cup applesauce, unsweetened (50)
  Noncaloric beverage

- **Evening Snack:** 195 calories
  - Evening Snack One
    or
  - Evening Snack Two

SATURDAY, Total calories, including snacks: 1,402

- **Breakfast:**   255 calories
  - Basic Breakfast One
    or
  - Basic Breakfast Two

- **Mid-morning Snack:**   102 calories
  - Mid-morning Snack One
    or
  - Mid-morning Snack Two

- **Lunch:**   352 calories
  - Basic Lunch One
    or
  - Basic Lunch Two

- **Mid-afternoon Fruit Snack:**   100 calories
  - Fruit Snack One
    or
  - Fruit Snack Two

- **Dinner:**   398 calories
  - Sweet & Sour Meatballs, Recipe #8 (218)
    ½ cup white rice (90)
    1 cup skim milk (90)

- **Evening Snack:**   195 calories
  - Evening Snack One
    or
  - Evening Snack Two

SUNDAY, Total calories, including snacks: 1,397

- **Breakfast:**   255 calories
  - Basic Breakfast One
    or
  - Basic Breakfast Two

- **Mid-morning Snack:** 102 calories
  - Mid-morning Snack One
    or
  - Mid-morning Snack Two

- **Lunch:** 352 calories
  - Basic Lunch One
    or
  - Basic Lunch Two

- **Mid-afternoon Fruit Snack:** 100 calories
  - Fruit Snack One
    or
  - Fruit Snack Two

- **Dinner:** 393 calories
  - * Chicken Paprika, Recipe #9 (188)
    1 ear corn, 5 inches long (70)
    1 cup French-style green beans (31)
    Salad:
      1 cup lettuce, chopped (9)
      2 slices tomato (14)
      1 tablespoon diet Italian dressing (6)
    ½ cup canned peaches, juice-packed (50)
    * with 1 tablespoon Home Granola, Recipe #1 (25)

- **Evening Snack:** 195 calories
  - Evening Snack One
    or
  - Evening Snack Two

···17···

Hip and Thigh Diet: Weeks 3 and 4

Only a few modifications have been incorporated into the Hip and Thigh diet for Weeks 3 and 4.

First, the daily calories decrease from 1,400 to 1,300. The missing calories are taken from the afternoon and evening snacks.

Second, Weeks 3 and 4 contain expanded options for the basic breakfasts, basic lunches, and evening snacks. Feel free to include them in your choices for the next two weeks.

MENUS FOR WEEKS 3 AND 4

MONDAY, Total calories, including snacks: 1,298

- **Breakfast:** 255 calories
  - **Basic Breakfast One**
    Cereal choices (1-ounce serving, 110 calories):
    Nabisco Shredded Wheat
    Kellogg's Frosted Mini-Wheats
    Kellogg's NutriGrain Wheat or Corn
    Post Grape Nuts
    Ralston Purina Almond Delight
    Ralston Purina Sun Flakes Crispy Wheat & Rice
    ³/₄ cup cooked oatmeal, sprinkled with cinnamon and
    low-calorie sweetener
  - *Plus*
    ¹/₂ cup skim milk (45)
    1 slice reduced-calorie bread, toasted (40)
    ¹/₂ tablespoon low-calorie margarine (25)

6 ounces low-calorie cranberry juice (35)
or
6 ounces vegetable juice cocktail (35)

OR

- **Basic Breakfast Two**
  8 ounces fruited, non-fat yogurt (any flavor), sweetened with aspartame (100)
  1 Nature Valley regular granola bar (Almond, Cinnamon, or Oats 'n Honey) (120)
  6 ounces low-calorie cranberry juice (35)
  or
  6 ounces vegetable juice cocktail (35)

OR

- **Basic Breakfast Three**
  1 oat bran waffle, frozen (120)
  Topping (heated):
    ½ cup applesauce, unsweetened (50)
    1 teaspoon low-calorie margarine (17)
    ½ teaspoon brown sugar (8)
    Sprinkle cinnamon
  ⅔ cup skim milk (60)

OR

- **Basic Breakfast Four**
  * 1 P-Nut Butter Muffin, Recipe #10 (130)
  6 ounces low-calorie cranberry juice (35)
  or
  6 ounces vegetable juice cocktail (35)
  1 cup skim milk (90)

- **Mid-morning Snack:** 102 calories
  - **Mid-morning Snack One**
  * 2 tablespoons Home Granola, Recipe #1 (50)
  2 tablespoons raisins (52)

OR

- **Mid-morning Snack Two**
  * Banana Snack Cake, Recipe #2 (50)
  1 teaspoon low-calorie margarine (17)

- **Lunch:**   352 calories
  - **Basic Lunch One**
  - * Pasta-Stuffed Tomato, Recipe #3 (204)
    1/2 cup fruited, non-fat yogurt (any flavor), sweetened
      with aspartame (50)
    1/2 medium banana (8 3/4 inches long) (50)
    4 saltines (48)
    Noncaloric beverage

  OR

  - **Basic Lunch Two**
  - * Chicken or Tuna or Turkey Salad Sandwich, Recipe #4
      (212)
    1/2 medium banana (8 3/4 inches long) (50)
    1 cup skim milk (90)

  OR

  - **Basic Lunch Three**
  - * Tex-Mex Tomato, Recipe #11 (200)
  - * Tortilla Chips, Recipe #5 (use 1 1/2 corn tortillas) (105)
    1/2 cup canned peaches, juice-packed (50)
    Sprinkle cinnamon on top of peaches
    Noncaloric beverage

  OR

  - **Basic Lunch Four**
    Whipped P-Nut Butter Sandwich:
      2 slices reduced-calorie oatmeal bread (80)
      1/2 medium banana (8 3/4 inches), sliced (50)
    * 2 tablespoons Whipped P-Nut Butter, from Recipe
      #10 (96)
    6 carrot strips (1/4-inch × 3-inch) (12)
    1 tablespoon raisins (26)
    1 cup skim milk (90)

- **Mid-afternoon Fruit Snack:**   50 calories
  - **Fruit Snack One**
    1/2 cup applesauce, unsweetened (50)

  OR

  - **Fruit Snack Two**
    1/2 fresh or canned pear, juice-packed (50)

**"NEW DINNER MENU OPTIONS APPEAR
AFTER SUNDAY MENU.**

- **Dinner:** 394 calories (" see menu options)
  Stouffer's Right Course Shrimp Primavera (240)
  Salad:
    Lettuce leaf (2)
    2 slices tomato (14)
    2 rings green pepper, 3-inch × ¼-inch thick (4)
    ½ cup cucumber, pared and diced (10)
    2 radishes, sliced (3)
    1 green onion, chopped (3)
  Creamy Italian Dressing:
    2 tablespoons non-fat yogurt (13)
    1 tablespoon diet Italian dressing (6)
  Garlic Bread:
    1 slice reduced-calorie bread (40)
    1 teaspoon low-calorie margarine (17)
    Sprinkling of powdered garlic or garlic salt
  ¼ cup applesauce, unsweetened (25), stir in
  ⅓ cup strawberries, sliced (17)
  Noncaloric beverage

- **Evening Snack:** 145 calories
  - **Evening Snack One**
  * Tortilla Chips, Recipe #5 (use 1¾ corn tortillas) (123)
    ¼ cup salsa (20)
    Noncaloric beverage

  OR

  - **Evening Snack Two**
    1¼ graham crackers (5 sections) (75)
    ¾ cup skim milk (68)

  OR

  - **Evening Snack Three**
    4 ounces fruited, non-fat yogurt (any flavor), sweetened
      with aspartame (50)
    * 1 tablespoon Whipped P-Nut Butter, from Recipe #10
      (48)
    (blend until smooth), add
    ⅓ cup banana, sliced (45)

TUESDAY, Total calories, including snacks: 1,307

- **Breakfast:** 255 calories
  - Basic Breakfast One
    or
  - Basic Breakfast Two
  - Basic Breakfast Three
    or
  - Basic Breakfast Four

- **Mid-morning Snack:** 102 calories
  - Mid-morning Snack One
    or
  - Mid-morning Snack Two

- **Lunch:** 352 calories
  - Basic Lunch One
    or
  - Basic Lunch Two
  - Basic Lunch Three
    or
  - Basic Lunch Four

- **Mid-afternoon Fruit Snack:** 50 calories
  - Fruit Snack One
    or
  - Fruit Snack Two

- **Dinner:** 403 calories
  - Chicken Fajitas, Recipe #6 (328)
    ½ cup canned peaches, juice-packed (50)
    ½ cup strawberries, sliced (25)
    Noncaloric beverage

- **Evening Snack:** 145 calories
  - Evening Snack One
    or
  - Evening Snack Two
    or
  - Evening Snack Three

WEDNESDAY, Total calories, including snacks: 1,305

- **Breakfast:** 255 calories
  - Basic Breakfast One
    or
  - Basic Breakfast Two
  - Basic Breakfast Three
    or
  - Basic Breakfast Four

- **Mid-morning Snack:**   102 calories
  - Mid-morning Snack One
    or
  - Mid-morning Snack Two

- **Lunch:**   352 calories
  - Basic Lunch One
    or
  - Basic Lunch Two
  - Basic Lunch Three
    or
  - Basic Lunch Four

- **Mid-afternoon Fruit Snack:**   50 calories
  - Fruit Snack One   *or*   • Fruit Snack Two

- **Dinner:**   401 calories
  Le Menu, 3-Cheese Stuffed Shells (280)
  Salad:
      1 slice pineapple, juice-packed, chopped (35)
      1 tablespoon raisins (26)
      1 teaspoon low-calorie mayonnaise (13)
      1 lettuce leaf (2)
  ³⁄₄ graham cracker, 3 sections (45)
  Noncaloric beverage

- **Evening Snack:**   145 calories
  - Evening Snack One
    or
  - Evening Snack Two
    or
  - Evening Snack Three

THURSDAY, Total calories, including snacks: 1,294

- **Breakfast:**   255 calories
  - Basic Breakfast One
    or
  - Basic Breakfast Two
  - Basic Breakfast Three
    or
  - Basic Breakfast Four

- **Mid-morning Snack:**   102 calories
  - Mid-morning Snack One
    or
  - Mid-morning Snack Two

- **Lunch:**   352 calories
  - Basic Lunch One
    or
  - Basic Lunch Two

  - Basic Lunch Three
    or
  - Basic Lunch Four

- **Mid-afternoon Fruit Snack:**   50 calories
  - Fruit Snack One
    or
  - Fruit Snack Two

- **Dinner:**   390 calories   (** see menu options)
  * Krab-Stuffed Potato, Recipe #7 (218)
    1 cup chopped broccoli, steamed (40)
    1 slice reduced-calorie bread (40)
    1 teaspoon low-calorie margarine (17)
    ½ canned peach, juice-packed (50)
  * with 1 tablespoon Home Granola, Recipe #1 (25)
    Noncaloric beverage

- **Evening Snack:**   145 calories
  - Evening Snack One
    or
  - Evening Snack Two
    or
  - Evening Snack Three

FRIDAY, Total calories, including snacks: 1,304
- **Breakfast:**   255 calories

  - Basic Breakfast One
    or
  - Basic Breakfast Two

  - Basic Breakfast Three
    or
  - Basic Breakfast Four

- **Mid-morning Snack:**   102 calories
  - Mid-morning Snack One
    or
  - Mid-morning Snack Two

- **Lunch:**   352 calories
  - Basic Lunch One
    or
  - Basic Lunch Two

  - Basic Lunch Three
    or
  - Basic Lunch Four

- **Mid-afternoon Fruit Snack:** 50 calories
  - Fruit Snack One
  or
  - Fruit Snack Two

- **Dinner:** 400 calories
  Weight Watchers Deluxe Combination Pizza (320)
  Salad:
  1 cup lettuce, chopped (9)
  1 slice tomato (7)
  1 tablespoon diet Italian dressing (6)
  Sprinkle dried basil
  Sprinkle 1 teaspoon Parmesan cheese (8)
  1/2 cup applesauce, unsweetened (50)
  Noncaloric beverage

- **Evening Snack:** 145 calories
  - Evening Snack One
  or
  - Evening Snack Two
  or
  - Evening Snack Three

SATURDAY, Total calories, including snacks: 1,302

- **Breakfast:** 255 calories
  - Basic Breakfast One
  or
  - Basic Breakfast Two
  - Basic Breakfast Three
  or
  - Basic Breakfast Four

- **Mid-morning Snack:** 102 calories
  - Mid-morning Snack One
  or
  - Mid-morning Snack Two

- **Lunch:** 352 calories
  - Basic Lunch One
  or
  - Basic Lunch Two
  - Basic Lunch Three
  or
  - Basic Lunch Four

- **Mid-afternoon Fruit Snack:** 50 calories
  - Fruit Snack One *or*
  - Fruit Snack Two

- **Dinner:**   398 calories (** see menu options)
  * Sweet & Sour Meatballs, Recipe #8 (218)
    ¹/₂ cup white rice (90)
    1 cup skim milk (90)

- **Evening Snack:**   145 calories
  - Evening Snack One
    or
  - Evening Snack Two
    or
  - Evening Snack Three

SUNDAY, Total calories, including snacks: 1,297

- **Breakfast:**   255 calories
  - Basic Breakfast One   • Basic Breakfast Three
    or   *or*
  - Basic Breakfast Two   • Basic Breakfast Four

- **Mid-morning Snack:**   102 calories
  - Mid-morning Snack One
    or
  - Mid-morning Snack Two

- **Lunch:**   352 calories
  - Basic Lunch One   • Basic Lunch Three
    or   *or*
  - Basic Lunch Two   • Basic Lunch Four

- **Mid-afternoon Fruit Snack:**   50 calories
  - Fruit Snack One
    or
  - Fruit Snack Two

- **Dinner:**   393 calories
  * Chicken Paprika, Recipe #9 (188)
    1 ear corn, 5 inches long (70)
    1 cup French-style green beans (31)
    Salad:
        1 cup lettuce, chopped (9)
        2 slices tomato (14)

1 tablespoon diet Italian dressing (6)
Sprinkle dried basil
1/2 cup canned peaches, juice-packed (50)
* with 1 tablespoon Home Granola, Recipe #1 (25)
Noncaloric beverage

• **Evening Snack:** 145 calories

  • Evening Snack One
    or
  • Evening Snack Two
    or
  • Evening Snack Three

**NEW DINNER MENU OPTIONS RECIPES ARE LISTED BELOW.

• **Monday Dinner Option:** 395 calories
  Booth Shrimp New Orleans (frozen dinner) (280)
  Salad:
    Lettuce leaf (2)
    2 slices tomato (14)
    2 rings green pepper, 3-inch × 1/4-inch thick (4)
    1/2 cup cucumber, pared and diced (10)
    2 radishes, sliced (3)
  Creamy Italian Dressing:
    2 tablespoons non-fat yogurt (13)
    1 tablespoon diet Italian dressing (6)
  1/2 cup canned peaches, juice-packed (50), top with
  1/2 tablespoon Home Granola, Recipe #1 (13)
  Noncaloric beverage

• **Saturday Dinner Option:** 402 calories
  * Meatball Stroganoff, Recipe #18 (272)
  1 cup chopped broccoli, steamed (40)
  1/2 cup applesauce, unsweetened (50)
  1 slice reduced-calorie bread (40)
  Noncaloric beverage

···18···
Hip and Thigh Diet: Weeks 5 and 6

:

By the start of the fifth week, you should be noticing significant changes in your hips and thighs.

On the scale you should have lost between 5 and 10 pounds, 7 pounds being the average. Seven pounds doesn't sound like much, but remember, if you've been exercising according to the routines in Chapters 23 and 24, you've put on some muscle weight. So your fat loss is more than your weight loss. You are changing your muscle-to-fat ratio for the better.

One of the best evaluations you can do is the tight-pants test. Try on the same pair of pants, a pair you had trouble squeezing into before you started the program, and notice how loose they fit. This is probably the single best way to determine the effectiveness, thus far, of the program. You'll be pleasantly surprised!

You should be even more enthused by the synergistic effects of the final two weeks. You'll be lowering your daily calories to 1,200, and you'll be raising the intensity of your exercise.

Keep your motivation high and your impatience low. Hot Hips and Fabulous Thighs will soon be yours.

MENUS FOR WEEKS 5 AND 6
·•·

MONDAY, Total calories, including snacks: 1,196

- **Breakfast:** 255 calories
  - **Basic Breakfast One**
    Cereal choices (1-ounce serving, 110 calories):
    Nabisco Shredded Wheat
    Kellogg's Frosted Mini-Wheats

Kellogg's NutriGrain Wheat or Corn
Post Grape Nuts
Ralston Purina Almond Delight
Ralston Purina Sun Flakes Crispy Wheat & Rice
3/4 cup cooked oatmeal, sprinkled with cinnamon and
    low-calorie sweetener

Plus
1/2 cup skim milk (45)
1 slice reduced-calorie bread, toasted (40)
1/2 tablespoon low-calorie margarine (25)
6 ounces low-calorie cranberry juice (35)
    or
6 ounces vegetable juice cocktail (35)

OR

- **Basic Breakfast Two**
  8 ounces fruited, non-fat yogurt (any flavor), sweetened
      with ˙aspartame (100)
  1 Nature Valley regular granola bar (Almond, Cinnamon,
      or Oats 'n Honey) (120)
  6 ounces low-calorie cranberry juice (35)
      or
  6 ounces vegetable juice cocktail (35)

OR

- **Basic Breakfast Three**
  1 oat bran waffle, frozen (120)
  Topping (heated):
      1/2 cup applesauce, unsweetened (50)
      1 teaspoon low-calorie margarine (17)
      1/2 teaspoon brown sugar (8)
      Sprinkle cinnamon
  2/3 cup skim milk (60)

OR

- **Basic Breakfast Four**
- 1 P-Nut Butter Muffin, Recipe #10 (130)
  6 ounces low-calorie cranberry juice (35)
      or
  6 ounces vegetable juice cocktail (35)
  1 cup skim milk (90)

OR

- **Basic Breakfast Five**
  ¹/₂ small grapefruit (40), broiled with
  1 teaspoon low-sugar raspberry jam (8)
* Country Omelet, Recipe #13 (150)
  1 slice reduced-calorie oatmeal bread (40)
  1 teaspoon low-calorie margarine (17)
  Noncaloric beverage

OR

- **Basic Breakfast Six**
  ¹/₂ cinnamon, raisin English muffin, toasted (75)
  ¹/₃ cup cottage cheese, 1% fat (57), mixed with
  ¹/₂ tablespoon raisins, snipped (13)
  Sprinkle cinnamon on top of cottage cheese
  1 slice canned pineapple, juice-packed (35)
  Noncaloric beverage

- **Mid-morning Snack:**   45 calories
* Spiced Tea, Recipe #14 (0)
  ³/₄ graham cracker (3 sections) (45)

- **Lunch:** 352 calories
  - **Basic Lunch One**
* Pasta-Stuffed Tomato, Recipe #3 (204)
  ¹/₂ cup fruited, non-fat yogurt (any flavor), sweetened
    with aspartame (50)
  ¹/₂ medium banana (8³/₄ inches long) (50)
  4 saltines (48)
  Noncaloric beverage

OR

- **Basic Lunch Two**
* Chicken or Tuna or Turkey Salad Sandwich, Recipe #4
    (212)
  ¹/₂ medium banana (8³/₄ inches long) (50)
  1 cup skim milk (90)

OR

- **Basic Lunch Three**
* Tex-Mex Tomato, Recipe #11 (200)
* Tortilla Chips, Recipe #5 (use 1 ¹/₂ corn tortillas) (105)

½ cup canned peaches, juice-packed (50)
Sprinkle cinnamon on top of peaches
Noncaloric beverage

OR

- **Basic Lunch Four**
  Whipped P-Nut Butter Sandwich:
  2 slices reduced-calorie oatmeal bread (80)
  ½ medium banana (8¾ inches), sliced (50)
  * 2 tablespoons Whipped P-Nut Butter, from Recipe
    #10 (96)
  6 carrot strips (¼-inch × 3-inch) (12)
  1 stalk celery (8 inches), cut into strips (7)
  1 tablespoon raisins (26)
  1 cup skim milk (90)

OR

- **Basic Lunch Five**
  * Fruit Sundae, Recipe #15 (205)
  * Cinnamon Crisps, Recipe #16 (131)
  6 carrot strips (¼ × 3) (12)
  1 stalk celery (8 inches), cut into strips (7)
  Noncaloric beverage

OR

- **Basic Lunch Six**
  * Spinach Salad in a Pocket, Recipe #17 (225)
  ½ cup fruited, non-fat yogurt (any flavor), sweetened
    with aspartame (50), stir in
  ½ medium banana (8¾ inches), sliced (50), topped
    with
  * 1 tablespoon Home Granola, Recipe #1 (25)

- **Mid-afternoon Fruit Snack:**   50 calories
  - **Fruit Snack One**
    ½ cup applesauce, unsweetened (50)

OR

- **Fruit Snack Two**
  ½ fresh pear or ½ cup canned pears, juice-packed (50)

**NEW DINNER MENU OPTIONS
APPEAR AFTER SUNDAY MENU

- **Dinner:**   394 calories   (** see menu options)
  Stouffer's Right Course Shrimp Primavera (240)
  Salad:
     Lettuce leaf (2)
     2 slices tomato (14)
     2 rings green pepper, 3-inch × 1/4-inch thick (4)
     1/2 cup cucumber, pared and diced (10)
     2 radishes, sliced (3)
  Creamy Italian Dressing:
     2 tablespoons non-fat yogurt (13)
     1 tablespoon diet Italian dressing (6)
  Garlic Bread:
     1 slice reduced-calorie bread (40)
     1 teaspoon low-calorie margarine (17)
     Sprinkling of powdered garlic or garlic salt
  1/4 cup applesauce, unsweetened (25), stir in
  1/3 cup strawberries, sliced (17)
  Noncaloric beverage

- **Evening Snack:** . 100 calories
  - **Evening Snack One**
  * Tortilla Chips, Recipe #5 (use 1 1/8 corn tortillas) (79)
    1/4 cup salsa (20)
    Noncaloric beverage

  OR

  - **Evening Snack Two**
    3/4 graham cracker (3 sections) (45)
    1/2 cup sugar-free cocoa (50)

  OR

  - **Evening Snack Three**
    4 ounces fruited, non-fat yogurt (any flavor), sweetened
      with aspartame (50)
  * 1 tablespoon Whipped P-Nut Butter, from Recipe #10
      (48)

  OR

  - **Evening Snack Four**
    1/2 cup ice milk (100)

TUESDAY, Total calories, including snacks: 1,205

- **Breakfast:** 255 calories
  - Basic Breakfast One
    or
  - Basic Breakfast Two
    or
  - Basic Breakfast Three

  - Basic Breakfast Four
    or
  - Basic Breakfast Five
    or
  - Basic Breakfast Six

- **Mid-morning Snack:** 45 calories
  * Spiced Tea, Recipe #14 (0)
    3/4 graham cracker (3 sections) (45)

- **Lunch:** 352 calories
  - Basic Lunch One
    or
  - Basic Lunch Two

  - Basic Lunch Three
    or
  - Basic Lunch Four

- **Mid-afternoon Fruit Snack:** 50 calories
  - Fruit Snack One
    or
  - Fruit Snack Two

- **Dinner:** 403 calories
  * Chicken Fajitas, Recipe #6 (328)
    1/2 cup canned peaches, juice-packed (50)
    1/2 cup strawberries, sliced (25)
    Noncaloric beverage

- **Evening Snack:** 100 calories
  - Evening Snack One
    or
  - Evening Snack Two

  - Evening Snack Three
    or
  - Evening Snack Four

WEDNESDAY, Total calories, including snacks: 1,203

- **Breakfast:** 255 calories
  - Basic Breakfast One
    or
  - Basic Breakfast Two
    or
  - Basic Breakfast Three

  - Basic Breakfast Four
    or
  - Basic Breakfast Five
    or
  - Basic Breakfast Six

- **Mid-morning Snack:** 45 calories
  * Spiced Tea, Recipe #14 (0)
  3/4 graham cracker (3 sections) (45)

- **Lunch:** 352 calories
  - Basic Lunch One
    or
  - Basic Lunch Two

  - Basic Lunch Three
    or
  - Basic Lunch Four

- **Mid-afternoon Fruit Snack:** 50 calories
  - Fruit Snack One
    or
  - Fruit Snack Two

- **Dinner:** 401 calories (** see menu options)
  Le Menu, 3-Cheese Stuffed Shells (280)
  Salad:
  1 slice pineapple, juice-packed, chopped (35)
  1 tablespoon raisins (26)
  1 teaspoon low-calorie mayonnaise (13)
  1 lettuce leaf (2)
  3/4 graham cracker, 3 sections (45)
  Noncaloric beverage

- **Evening Snack:** 100 calories
  - Evening Snack One
    or
  - Evening Snack Two

  - Evening Snack Three
    or
  - Evening Snack Four

THURSDAY, Total calories, including snacks: 1,192

- **Breakfast:** 255 calories
  - Basic Breakfast One
    or
  - Basic Breakfast Two
    or
  - Basic Breakfast Three

  - Basic Breakfast Four
    or
  - Basic Breakfast Five
    or
  - Basic Breakfast Six

- **Mid-morning Snack:** 45 calories
  * Spiced Tea, Recipe #14 (0)
  3/4 graham cracker (3 sections) (45)

- **Lunch:**   352 calories
  - Basic Lunch One
    or
  - Basic Lunch Two
  - Basic Lunch Three
    or
  - Basic Lunch Four

- **Mid-afternoon Fruit Snack:**   50 calories
  - Fruit Snack One
    or
  - Fruit Snack Two

- **Dinner:**   390 calories   (** see menu options)
  * Krab-Stuffed Potato, Recipe #7 (218)
    1 cup chopped broccoli, steamed (40)
    1 slice reduced-calorie bread (40)
    1 teaspoon low-calorie margarine (17)
    1/2 canned peach, juice-packed (50)
  *   with 1 tablespoon Home Granola, Recipe #1 (25)
    Noncaloric beverage

- **Evening Snack:**   100 calories
  - Evening Snack One
    or
  - Evening Snack Two
  - Evening Snack Three
    or
  - Evening Snack Four

FRIDAY, Total calories, including snacks: 1,202

- **Breakfast:**   255 calories
  - Basic Breakfast One
    or
  - Basic Breakfast Two
    or
  - Basic Breakfast Three
  - Basic Breakfast Four
    or
  - Basic Breakfast Five
    or
  - Basic Breakfast Six

- **Mid-morning Snack:**   45 calories
  * Spiced Tea, Recipe #14 (0)
    3/4 graham cracker (3 sections) (45)

- **Lunch:**   352 calories
  - Basic Lunch One
    or
  - Basic Lunch Two
  - Basic Lunch Three
    or
  - Basic Lunch Four

- **Mid-afternoon Fruit Snack:**   50 calories
  - Fruit Snack One
    or
  - Fruit Snack Two

- **Dinner:**   400 calories   (** see menu options)
  Weight Watchers Deluxe Combination Pizza (320)
  Salad:
  > 1 cup lettuce, chopped (9)
  > 1 slice tomato (7)
  > 1 tablespoon diet Italian dressing (6)
  > Sprinkle dried basil
  > Sprinkle 1 teaspoon Parmesan cheese (8)
  1/2 cup applesauce, unsweetened (50)
  Noncaloric beverage

- **Evening Snack:**   100 calories
  - Evening Snack One   • Evening Snack Three
    or   *or*
  - Evening Snack Two   • Evening Snack Four

SATURDAY, Total calories, including snacks: 1,200

- **Breakfast:**   255 calories
  - Basic Breakfast One   • Basic Breakfast Four
    or   *or*
  - Basic Breakfast Two   • Basic Breakfast Five
    or   *or*
  - Basic Breakfast Three   • Basic Breakfast Six

- **Mid-morning Snack:**   45 calories
  - Spiced Tea, Recipe #14 (0)
    3/4 graham cracker (3 sections) (45)

- **Lunch:**   352 calories
  - Basic Lunch One   • Basic Lunch Three
    or   *or*
  - Basic Lunch Two   • Basic Lunch Four

- **Mid-afternoon Fruit Snack:**   50 calories
  - Fruit Snack One   *or*   • Fruit Snack Two

- **Dinner:** 398 calories (** see menu options)
- * Sweet & Sour Meatballs, Recipe #8 (218)
  1/2 cup white rice (90)
  1 cup skim milk (90)

- **Evening Snack:** 100 calories
  - Evening Snack One
    or
  - Evening Snack Two

  - Evening Snack Three
    or
  - Evening Snack Four

SUNDAY, Total calories, including snacks: 1,195

- **Breakfast:** 255 calories
  - Basic Breakfast One
    or
  - Basic Breakfast Two
    or
  - Basic Breakfast Three

  - Basic Breakfast Four
    or
  - Basic Breakfast Five
    or
  - Basic Breakfast Six

- **Mid-morning Snack:** 45 calories
  * Spiced Tea, Recipe #14 (0)
  3/4 graham cracker (3 sections) (45)

- **Lunch:** 352 calories
  - Basic Lunch One
    or
  - Basic Lunch Two

  - Basic Lunch Three
    or
  - Basic Lunch Four

- **Mid-afternoon Fruit Snack:** 50 calories
  - Fruit Snack One *or*
  - Fruit Snack Two

- **Dinner:** 393 calories
  * Chicken Paprika, Recipe #9 (188)
    1 ear corn, 5 inches long (70)
    1 cup French-style green beans (31)
    Salad:
    1 cup lettuce, chopped (9)
    2 slices tomato (14)
    1 tablespoon diet Italian dressing (6)
    Sprinkle dried basil
    1/2 cup canned peaches, juice-packed (50)
  * with 1 tablespoon Home Granola, Recipe #1 (25)

- **Evening Snack:**   100 calories
  - Evening Snack One   • Evening Snack Three
    or   *or*
  - Evening Snack Two   • Evening Snack Four

"NEW DINNER MENU OPTIONS RECIPES ARE LISTED BELOW.

- **Monday Dinner Option:**   445 calories

  Booth Shrimp New Orleans (frozen dinner) (280)
  Salad:
  1 slice canned pineapple, juice-packed (35)
  2 dates, chopped (40)
  Sprinkle ginger
  1 cup skim milk (90)

- **Wednesday Dinner Option:**   400 calories

  Weight Watchers Broccoli & Cheese Baked Potato (280)
  2 slices tomato (14)
  1 tablespoon diet Italian dressing (6)
  Sprinkle dried basil
  ½ cinnamon, raisin English muffin, toasted (75)
  ½ cup strawberries, sliced (25)
  Noncaloric beverage

- **Thursday Dinner Option:**   389 calories

  * Homestyle Eggplant, Recipe #12 (250)
  1 cup French-style green beans (31)
  Salad:
  Lettuce leaf (2)
  2 slices tomato (14)
  2 rings green pepper, 3-inch × ¼-inch thick (4)
  2 radishes, sliced (3)
  1 green onion, chopped (3)
  Creamy Italian Dressing:
  2 tablespoons non-fat yogurt (13)
  1 tablespoon diet Italian dressing (6)
  ½ cup canned peaches, juice-packed (50), top with
  * ½ tablespoon Home Granola, Recipe #1 (13)
  Noncaloric beverage

- **Friday Dinner Option:** 401 calories

  Lean Cuisine, Filet of Fish Jardiniere with Souffléed
    Potatoes (280)
  Salad:
    1 slice pineapple, juice-packed (35)
    1 tablespoon raisins (26)
    1 teaspoon low-calorie mayonnaise (13)
    1 lettuce leaf (2)
  ³/₄ graham cracker (3 sections) (45)
  Noncaloric beverage

- **Saturday Dinner Option:** 402 calories

  * Meatball Stroganoff, Recipe #18 (272)
    1 cup chopped broccoli, steamed (40)
    ¹/₂ cup applesauce, unsweetened (50)
    1 slice reduced-calorie bread (40)
    Noncaloric beverage

···19···

Hot and Fabulous Recipes

All the recipes in this chapter are nutritious and delicious. Plus, they require only a moderate amount of preparation time.

The recipes are numbered consecutively to correspond with their appearance in the text.

● *Recipe #1*

HOME GRANOLA

1   tablespoon low-calorie margarine
1   tablespoon molasses
1/2 teaspoon vanilla extract
1/4 teaspoon ground cinnamon
1   cup rolled oats, uncooked

Preheat oven to 300 degrees. Place the margarine and molasses in a 1-quart micro-proof casserole dish; microwave on 50% power for 30 seconds or until margarine is melted. Stir in the vanilla and cinnamon; add the oats and toss to cover evenly. Bake at 300 degrees for 20 to 25 minutes or until lightly browned. Stir every 10 minutes.

Allow to cool; store in glass jar. This crunchy treat is good for quick snacks by itself, combined with fresh or dried fruit, stirred into yogurt, or as a topping on countless foods.

YIELD: 1 cup
CALORIES: 25 per tablespoon

● *Recipe #2*

BANANA SNACK CAKE
● ● ●

1 ¼ cups quick-cooking oats, uncooked
½ cup raisins
½ cup chopped dates
¼ cup whole bran cereal
½ cup unsweetened crushed pineapple, undrained
1 large over-ripe banana (9 ¾ inches long)
¼ cup frozen egg substitute (thawed)
2 tablespoons low-calorie margarine, melted
1 ½ teaspoons baking powder
½ teaspoon ground cinnamon
1 teaspoon vanilla extract
¼ teaspoon salt
   Butter-flavor cooking spray

Preheat oven to 350 degrees. Combine oats, raisins, dates, and cereal in a large bowl; set aside. Mix the remaining ingredients, except cooking spray, in container of blender or food processor; process until smooth. Add banana mixture to dry ingredients, stirring until well blended.

Treat muffin pan with cooking spray. Spoon batter evenly into muffin pan. Bake at 350 degrees for 30 to 35 minutes. (Snack cake does not rise during baking.)

YIELD: 1 dozen muffins
CALORIES: 85 per muffin
Also: Add 1 teaspoon low-calorie margarine (17) to each muffin.

● *Recipe #3*

PASTA-STUFFED TOMATO
— • • • —

½   cup corkscrew or plain macaroni, uncooked
¼   cup early green peas, frozen
1   small carrot (5 inches long), sliced
1   small green onion, chopped
½   cup celery, sliced
1   teaspoon dried parsley
¼   cup diet Italian dressing
2   tablespoons plain, non-fat yogurt
    Pinch dried basil
    Sprinkle garlic powder
    Pepper to taste
1   teaspoon Parmesan cheese
2   medium tomatoes (3-inch diameter)

Cook macaroni according to directions, omitting salt;
drain. Cook peas briefly, just to tender stage. Combine
all ingredients, except tomato; toss well. Chill at least
one hour.

Place tomatoes stem-end down. Cut each tomato into
six wedges (be sure to cut to, but *not* through base of
tomato). Spread wedges slightly apart; spoon half of
pasta mixture into each tomato.

YIELD: 2 servings
CALORIES: 204 per serving

● *Recipe #4*

CHICKEN OR TUNA OR TURKEY
SALAD SANDWICH
— • • • —

1   (6¾-ounce) can of white meat chicken, tuna
     (water-packed) or white meat turkey, drained
1   hard-boiled egg, chopped
1   tablespoon reduced-calorie mayonnaise

$^1/_2$ cup celery, sliced
3   dill pickle spears (6 inches long), chopped
2   tablespoons diet Italian dressing
$^1/_4$ teaspoon celery seed
     Sprinkle garlic powder or garlic salt
     Sprinkle pepper

Flake selected meat in a medium-size mixing bowl. Add remaining ingredients and toss to mix well. Refrigerate at least one hour to allow flavors to blend.

YIELD: 3 servings
CALORIES: 123 per serving

ASSEMBLE SANDWICH: (212 calories)

2   slices reduced-calorie bread
$^1/_3$ salad sandwich mixture
1   slice tomato
1   lettuce leaf

• **Recipe #5**

TORTILLA CHIPS
— • • • —

1   corn tortilla (1 ounce)
     Salt (optional)

Preheat oven to 400 degrees. Cut the tortilla into 8 pie-shaped wedges. Spread the pieces on a nonstick baking sheet and lightly sprinkle with salt (optional).

Bake at 400 degrees for about 5 to 8 minutes (be careful not to let chips burn). Remove from the oven and turn each wedge with tongs or a pancake turner. Bake for 3 to 4 minutes. Cool on a paper towel.

YIELD: 8 chips
CALORIES: 70
NOTE: Prepare the number of tortillas as directed in menu.

• **Recipe #6**

CHICKEN FAJITAS
— • • —

Butter-flavor cooking spray
$\frac{1}{2}$ tablespoon low-calorie margarine
4   ounces (raw weight) boneless, skinless chicken
    strips
$\frac{1}{4}$ cup onion slices
$\frac{1}{4}$ cup green pepper strips
$\frac{1}{4}$ cup sweet red pepper strips
$\frac{1}{4}$ cup julienne carrots (3-inch)
$\frac{1}{4}$ cup julienne zucchini (3-inch)
1   flour tortilla (6-inch)
1   tablespoon Worcestershire sauce
$\frac{1}{4}$ fresh lemon wedge

Treat nonstick skillet with cooking spray; add margarine
and melt. Brown chicken in skillet until no longer pink
at center. Remove chicken and drain on paper toweling.
Add all the vegetable slices and sauté until tender.
Return chicken to skillet and heat thoroughly. Just
before serving, heat flour tortilla; add Worcestershire
sauce to chicken/vegetable mixture and toss, then
squeeze on lemon and toss again.

Place heated tortilla on a dinner plate; top with
chicken/vegetable mixture on one side and fold over.
Serve immediately.

YIELD: 1 serving
CALORIES: 328

• *Recipe #7*

CRAB-STUFFED POTATO
• • •

1   small baking potato (4 1/2 ounces), scrubbed
     Butter-flavor cooking spray
2   ounces chopped imitation crab meat
     Juice of 1/4 fresh lemon
1/4   cup low-fat (1%) cottage cheese, whipped with
      mixer until smooth
2   tablespoons green onion, sliced (include green tops)
2   tablespoons red bell pepper, chopped
1   tablespoon non-fat plain yogurt
     Salt and pepper to taste
1/2   teaspoon sour-cream and butter-flavor sprinkles
     Paprika

Pierce potato with fork tines several times. Spray a small amount of cooking spray on potato; rub potato with hands to distribute evenly. Place on paper towel and microwave on high for 4 to 5 minutes; let stand 2 minutes.

Allow potato to cool slightly; cut in half lengthwise; scoop pulp from each half into small bowl, leaving a 1/2-inch thick shell; set aside.

Mash potato; add remaining ingredients, except paprika, and mix until smooth. Spoon mixture into shells and sprinkle with paprika.

Place stuffed potato on a plate and microwave on high 1 to 2 minutes, or until heated through.

YIELD: 1 serving
CALORIES: 218

• *Recipe #8*

SWEET & SOUR MEATBALLS
• • •

6   freezer turkey meatballs (recipe to follow)
1   8-ounce can chunk pineapple, juice-packed
        (reserve 1/4 cup juice)
1/4   cup water
1   tablespoon cider vinegar
1/2   medium green pepper (3-inch diameter), cut into
        strips
1 1/2   teaspoons cornstarch
1 1/2   teaspoons brown sugar
1   tablespoon low-sodium soy sauce

Combine meatballs, reserved pineapple juice, water, and
vinegar; heat to boiling. Cover; simmer 15 minutes,
turning meatballs as they cook. Add green pepper;
simmer an additional 5 minutes. Blend cornstarch,
brown sugar, and soy sauce; add to meatball mixture.
Cook and stir until clear and thickened. Stir in
pineapple; heat thoroughly. Divide evenly and serve
over hot cooked white rice.

YIELD: 2 servings
CALORIES: 218 per serving

FREEZER TURKEY MEATBALLS

1   egg
1/4   cup skim milk
1   pound ground turkey
2   tablespoons dried bread crumbs
1/4   teaspoon salt
1/8   teaspoon pepper
1/4   teaspoon dried thyme
1   tablespoon Worcestershire sauce

Heat oven to 400 degrees. Blend egg and milk in
medium bowl. Stir in remaining ingredients; mix well.
Shape into twelve 1 1/2-inch balls. Place in non-stick
13 × 9-inch pan. Bake at 400 degrees for 15 to 20
minutes or until lightly browned. Cool 5 minutes; place

meatballs on cookie sheet. Freeze uncovered for 45 minutes. Place partially frozen meatballs into 2 freezer-proof containers or freezer bags; label (6 meatballs and date). Meatballs can be frozen up to 3 months.

Microwave Directions: Prepare meatballs as directed above. Place meatballs in 2-quart micro-safe baking dish. Arrange meatballs around outside edge of dish, leaving the center empty. Microwave 4 minutes on high. Turn meatballs over; continue cooking on high for 4 minutes or until meat reaches desired doneness. Cool 5 minutes; freeze as instructed above.

YIELD: 12 meatballs   **CALORIES:**   43 per meatball

● *Recipe #9*

CHICKEN PAPRIKA
—————————●●●—————————

2   chicken breast halves, boned and skinned (8 ounces raw weight)
      Dash salt, optional
      Pepper to taste
½   tablespoon paprika
¼   cup onion, finely chopped
2   tablespoons dry white wine
½   tablespoon all-purpose flour
½   cup non-fat yogurt

Place chicken in a micro-safe casserole dish. Sprinkle with seasonings; add onion and wine and cover. Microwave on high (100% power) for 8 minutes; turn chicken over and continue cooking on high for 7 to 10 more minutes, or until juices run clear. Remove chicken and drain on paper toweling. Skim fat from pan drippings. Stir flour into yogurt and blend into casserole. Microwave 1½ to 2½ minutes on medium heat (50% power). Divide sauce evenly and pour over each chicken breast half.

YIELD: 2 servings   **CALORIES:**   188 per serving

• *Recipe #10*

P-NUT BUTTER MUFFINS
• • •

Butter-flavor cooking spray
3   tablespoons Whipped P-Nut Butter (recipe to follow)
1   large egg
1   cup skim milk
2   tablespoons vegetable oil
2   cups raisin bran cereal
1   cup all-purpose flour, spooned into cup
1/3 cup brown sugar
1/2 teaspoon salt
2   teaspoons baking powder

Preheat oven to 400 degrees; treat muffin pan with cooking spray and set aside. Blend Whipped P-Nut Butter, egg, milk, and oil together in a medium mixing bowl; add raisin bran. Let stand 10 minutes; stir.

Mix remaining ingredients together in a large bowl; add cereal mixture all at once to dry ingredients. Stir just until moistened. Spoon evenly into muffin pan. Bake at 400 degrees for 20 to 25 minutes or until fork inserted in center comes out clean.

YIELD: 12 muffins
CALORIES: 130 per muffin

WHIPPED P-NUT BUTTER

4 1/2   ounces dry-roasted, unseasoned peanuts **
1/2 to 2/3   cup cold water
1/2 to 1   package aspartame (optional)

Puree peanuts to a paste in the workbowl of a food processor or blender container. Gradually add enough cold water until P-Nut Butter is the consistency of jam (be careful not to let it become too thin). If desired, add sweetener.

Pack into clean jar and store in refrigerator until ready to use. (HINT: Do not assemble Whipped P-Nut Butter Sandwich until mealtime. Keep P-Nut Butter refrigerated in small container.)

YIELD: 16 tablespoons
CALORIES: 48 per tablespoon
"NOTE: You may find seasoned, dry-roasted peanuts more flavorful for sandwiches.

• *Recipe #11*

TEX-MEX TOMATO
• • •

Dressing:
   2   tablespoons olive or vegetable oil
   2   tablespoons diet Italian dressing
   4   cloves garlic, minced
   1   teaspoon hot-pepper sauce
   $1/2$ teaspoon pepper
   $1/4$ teaspoon salt (optional)
1   can (about 16 ounces) black beans, drained
1   4-ounce can chopped green chili peppers, drained
$1/3$ cup green onion, thinly sliced
4   medium tomatoes (3-inch diameter)

Mix dressing ingredients in a large bowl; add remaining ingredients. Stir gently to mix and coat; set aside.

Place tomatoes stem end down. Cut each tomato into six wedges (be sure to cut to, but *not* through, base of tomato). Spread wedges slightly apart; spoon half of bean mixture into each tomato.

YIELD: 4 stuffed tomatoes
CALORIES: 200 per stuffed tomato

• *Recipe #12*

HOME-STYLE EGGPLANT
• • •

1   pound eggplant, sliced
½   cup water
     Butter-flavor cooking spray
½   cup chopped onion
5   medium mushrooms, sliced
1   (14½-ounce) can Italian-style stewed tomatoes
       (with basil, garlic, and oregano)
¼   cup chopped parsley
½   teaspoon thyme
⅛   teaspoon garlic powder or garlic salt
     Dash pepper
8   slices reduced-calorie Italian bread
4   ounces part-skim mozzarella cheese, grated
¼   cup grated Parmesan cheese

Preheat oven to 400 degrees. Place eggplant slices and
½ cup water in skillet. Cook until tender, about 10
minutes; drain, reserving liquid. Treat skillet with
cooking spray; cook onion and mushrooms until onion
is soft. Stir in tomatoes, parsley, herbs, garlic powder,
and pepper. Drain, reserving liquid; add to reserved
eggplant liquid.

  Treat an 8-inch square baking dish with cooking
spray; line with half the bread. Top with half the
eggplant and half the tomato mixture. Top with half the
mozzarella and sprinkle with half the Parmesan. Repeat
bread, eggplant, and tomato layers. Pour reserved liquid
over the layers. Cover and bake at 450 degrees and
sprinkle with remaining cheese. Continue baking
uncovered 5 minutes or until cheese melts. Let stand 5
minutes. Cut into 4 squares and serve.

YIELD: 4 servings
CALORIES: 250 per serving

● *Recipe #13*

COUNTRY OMELET
● ● ●

1   large egg
1   tablespoon water
   Salt and pepper to taste
   Pinch dried thyme
   Pinch dried basil
   Butter-flavor cooking spray
1   tablespoon finely chopped onion
2   tablespoons chopped green pepper
1   slice (1 ounce) reduced-calorie sharp cheddar
    cheese (50)
2   slices tomato, chopped

Place egg and water in a bowl and whisk just enough to blend together. Do not overbeat. Add a pinch of salt, pepper, and herbs. Set aside.

Treat a 6- or 7-inch nonstick skillet with cooking spray and heat. Add onion and green pepper; cook and stir until the vegetables are tender. Pour egg over vegetables, tilting pan to distribute evenly. As mixture begins to cook, gently lift edge with a spatula and tilt pan to allow liquid egg to flow underneath. Continue until there is no more liquid egg. Divide the cheese slice in half. Place half the cheese on one side of the omelet, top with tomato; fold omelet in half. Place remaining cheese on omelet; cover skillet and remove from heat. When cheese is softened (about 1 minute), slide onto a warm plate.

YIELD: 1 serving
CALORIES: 150

• *Recipe #14*

SPICED TEA
• • •

1   cup hot water
1/2 teaspoon grated orange peel
1/4 teaspoon grated lemon peel
2   whole cloves
1/2 cinnamon stick
1   decaf tea bag

Combine water, orange peel, lemon peel, and spices in a small casserole dish. Cover; microwave on high 3 to 5 minutes, or until boiling. Remove from oven; immediately add tea bag and let steep 2 to 3 minutes. Serve hot or chilled.

YIELD: 1 serving   **CALORIES:** 0

• *Recipe #15*

FRUIT SUNDAE
• • •

1/2 cup cottage cheese (1% fat)
2   teaspoons low-sugar orange marmalade
    Sprinkle cinnamon
1/2 cup canned fruit cocktail, juice-packed
1/2 cup strawberries, sliced
    Sprinkle ground nutmeg
1   cup torn lettuce or spinach leaves
1   tablespoon Home Granola, from Recipe #1

Mix cottage cheese, marmalade, and cinnamon together in a small dish and set aside. Combine fruit cocktail and strawberries together and sprinkle with nutmeg in a small dish and set aside.

Line a salad plate with lettuce or spinach leaves; place cottage cheese in the center and top with mixed fruit. Top with Home Granola and enjoy.

HINT: Brown Baggers should carry the cottage cheese mixture and the fruit mixture separately in small containers and lettuce or spinach in a sandwich bag. Assemble at mealtime.

YIELD: 1 serving   **CALORIES:** 205

• *Recipe #16*

CINNAMON CRISPS
• • •

Butter-flavor cooking spray
1   teaspoon low-calorie margarine
1   flour tortilla (6-inch diameter)
1   package low-calorie sweetener
Sprinkle cinnamon

Heat oven to 400 degrees. Treat nonstick baking sheet with cooking spray; set aside.

Spread low-calorie margarine evenly on flour tortilla and cut into 8 wedges. Place wedges, margarine-side up, on baking sheet. Cook at 400 degrees until margarine has melted and chips are light brown, 3 to 5 minutes.

Combine low-calorie sweetener and cinnamon in a plastic bag; add warm chips and shake to coat. Serve warm or allow to cool and store in sandwich bag for mealtime.

YIELD: 1 serving (8 crisps)
CALORIES: 131

• *Recipe #17*

SPINACH SALAD IN A POCKET
• • •

1   hard-boiled egg
1/2   cup shredded zucchini, uncooked
1/4   cup shredded carrot
1/4   cup plain, non-fat yogurt
1 1/2   tablespoons diet Italian dressing
1   whole wheat pita (4-inch diameter)
1   cup fresh spinach leaves
1   teaspoon real bacon bits, canned

Chop boiled egg and combine with zucchini and carrot; toss and set aside. Mix yogurt and dressing together in a measuring cup. Add yogurt mixture to egg and vegetables; toss to coat evenly.

Cut pita pocket in half. Line each half with spinach leaves and stuff each pocket half with ½ the egg and vegetable mixture. Sprinkle bacon bits on each sandwich.

HINT: Brown Baggers should assemble sandwich at mealtime. Carry the divided pita, spinach, and bacon bits in a sandwich bag, the yogurt dressing in a separate container from the egg and vegetable mixture. At mealtime, combine the yogurt dressing with the egg and vegetable mixture and assemble as directed above.

YIELD: 1 serving   **CALORIES:** 225

- *Recipe #18*

MEATBALL STROGANOFF
• • •

6   Freezer Meatballs (from Recipe #8)
1   (7 ½-ounce) can semi-condensed cream of
      mushroom soup
1   (2 ½-ounce) can sliced mushrooms, drained
½   teaspoon catsup
1   teaspoon Worcestershire sauce
3   ounces (dry weight) noodles
½   tablespoon flour
½   teaspoon chopped chives
¼   cup plain non-fat yogurt

Combine first 5 ingredients in a medium saucepan; heat to boiling. Cover and simmer for about 20 minutes, turning meatballs as they cook.

While meatballs cook: prepare noodles according to package directions. Stir flour and chives into yogurt in a measuring cup. After 20 minutes, remove meatballs from heat and stir yogurt mixture into meatballs.

Drain noodles and divide evenly into 3 servings; top each with ⅓ meatball stroganoff.

YIELD: 3 servings
CALORIES: 272 per serving

···20···

Shopping Lists

:

The first shopping list tells you everything you need to prepare the menus and recipes for Week 1. Week 2 is a repeat of the first week. Shopping lists for Weeks 3, 4, 5, and 6 follow Weeks 1 and 2.

Staples, packaged goods, and frozen products last for many weeks and can be purchased in quantities greater than those indicated. Some produce should not be bought more than a week in advance, and foods such as poultry, meat, and especially fish may not remain fresh for even a few days unless you freeze them. When you bring your groceries home, keep perishability in mind so you can freeze items if necessary. Check supplies at the end of the first week.

Quantities needed for items marked with an asterisk (*) will depend on your specific selections for Basic Breakfasts, Basic Lunches, and Snacks. Review the selections and make adjustments accordingly. You may vary these selections from week to week.

WEEKS 1 AND 2
···

HAVE ON HAND: STAPLES
* non-caloric beverages (water, coffee, tea, diet soft drinks)
* reduced-calorie bread (40 calories per slice)
* cereal (110 calories per ounce), choose from:
Nabisco Shredded Wheat
Kellogg's Frosted Mini-Wheats
Kellogg's NutriGrain Wheat or Corn
Oatmeal (not individual packages)
Post Grape Nuts
Ralston Purina Almond Delight
Ralston Purina Sun Flakes
Crispy Wheat & Rice

111

* Nature Valley Granola Bars (Almond, Cinnamon, or Oats 'n Honey)
* graham crackers

  low-calorie margarine (50 calories per tablespoon)

  low-calorie mayonnaise (40 calories per tablespoon)

  Parmesan cheese

  raisins

  salt
* saltine crackers

  skim milk

  vegetable cooking spray (butter flavor)

HERBS, SPICES, SEASONINGS

  dried basil
* celery seed

  cinnamon

  garlic powder

  garlic salt (optional)

  paprika
* dried parsley

  dried thyme

  vanilla

  Worcestershire sauce

MEAT, FISH, POULTRY

  chicken breast halves (raw weight 4 ounces each), 3
* canned white meat chicken (2-ounce serving)

  imitation crab meat, 2 ounces

  ground turkey, 1 pound
* canned turkey, white meat (2-ounce serving)
* canned tuna, water-packed (2-ounce serving)

FROZEN DINNERS

  Le Menu Light Style: 3-Cheese Stuffed Shells, 1

  Weight Watchers: Deluxe Combination Pizza, 1

  Stouffer's Right Course Shrimp Primavera, 1

DAIRY PRODUCTS

* plain yogurt, non-fat, 8 ounces
* fruited yogurt, non-fat, sweetened with aspartame (100 calories per 8 ounces)

BREADS, CEREALS

* 100% whole bran cereal
* corn tortillas

  dried bread crumbs, 2 tablespoons

  flour tortilla, (8-inch diameter), 1
* macaroni (corkscrew or plain)

  white rice

FRUITS, VEGETABLES, JUICES

* apple, medium (3-inch diameter)

  applesauce, unsweetened, 1 cup

  bananas, medium (8¾ inches long), 4
* banana, ripe, large (9¾ inches long), 1

  broccoli, fresh or frozen, 1 cup
* carrots
* celery

  corn on the cob (5 inches long), fresh or frozen, 1 ear

* cranberry juice cocktail, low-calorie
* cucumber
* dates
* dill pickle spears (6 inches long)
* green beans, French-style, fresh or frozen, 1 cup
* green onion, 1
* green peas, early, frozen
green pepper, medium (3-inch diameter), 1
lettuce, 1 large head
lemon, fresh, 1 large
* mushrooms, fresh, 5
onion, white, 1 medium
canned peaches, juice-packed, 1
* canned pineapple slices, juice-packed, 1
canned pineapple crushed, juice-packed, 4 ounces
canned pineapple chunks, juice-packed, 8 ounces
potato, small (2 1/2-inch diameter, 4 1/2 ounces), 1

radish, 2
* salsa, canned in jars, 1
sweet red pepper, medium (3-inch diameter), 1
* strawberries (fresh or frozen without sugar), 1 cup
* tomatoe, medium (3-inch diameter), 1
* vegetable juice cocktail
zucchini, 1/4 cup

MISCELLANEOUS
all-purpose flour, 1/2 tablespoon
baking powder
brown sugar
cider vinegar, 1 tablespoon
cornstarch
diet Italian dressing (6 calories per tablespoon)
dry white wine, 1/2 cup
egg substitute, frozen
* molasses
low-sodium soy sauce
sour-cream and butter-flavor sprinkles

WEEKS 3 AND 4
—————•••—————

HAVE ON HAND: STAPLES
* non-caloric beverages (water, coffee, tea, diet soft drinks)
* reduced-calorie bread (40 calories per slice)
* cereal (110 calories per ounce), choose from:
Nabisco Shredded Wheat
Kellogg's Frosted Mini-Wheats
Kellogg's NutriGrain Wheat or Corn

Oatmeal (not individual packages)
Post Grape Nuts
Ralston Purina Almond Delight
Ralston Purina Sun Flakes
Crispy Wheat & Rice
* Nature Valley Granola Bars (Almond, Cinnamon, or Oats 'n Honey)
* graham crackers

low-calorie margarine (50 calories per tablespoon)
low-calorie mayonnaise (40 calories per tablespoon)
Parmesan cheese
raisins
salt
* saltine crackers
skim milk
vegetable cooking spray (butter flavor)
* vegetable cooking oil

HERBS, SPICES, SEASONINGS

dried basil
* celery seed
cinnamon
* garlic cloves, 4
garlic powder
garlic salt (optional)
* green chili peppers, chopped (4-ounce can)
* hot-pepper sauce
paprika
* dried parsley
dried thyme
vanilla
Worcestershire sauce

MEAT, FISH, POULTRY

chicken breast halves (raw weight 4 ounces each), 3
* canned white meat chicken (2-ounce serving)
imitation crab meat, 2 ounces
* eggs
* peanuts, dry-roasted, 4 1/2 ounces
ground turkey, 1 pound

* canned turkey, white meat (2-ounce serving)
* canned tuna, water-packed (2-ounce serving)

FROZEN DINNERS

Le Menu Light Style: 3-Cheese Stuffed Shells, 1
Weight Watchers: Deluxe Combination Pizza, 1
Stouffer's Right Course Shrimp Primavera, 1
* Booth: Shrimp New Orleans, 1

DAIRY PRODUCTS

* part-skim mozzarella cheese, 4 ounces
* plain yogurt, non-fat, 8 ounces
* fruited yogurt, non-fat, sweetened with aspartame (100 calories per 8 ounces)

BREADS, CEREALS

* 100% whole bran cereal
* corn tortillas
dried bread crumbs, 2 tablespoons
flour tortilla, (6-inch diameter), 1
* macaroni (corkscrew or plain)
* raisin bran cereal, 2 cups
white rice
* reduced-calorie Italian bread, 40 calories/slice, 4 slices
* oat bran waffles (frozen), 120 calories/waffle

FRUITS, VEGETABLES, JUICES

* apple, medium (3-inch diameter)
applesauce, unsweetened, 1 cup
bananas, medium (8 3/4 inches long), 4
* banana, ripe, large (9 3/4 inches long), 1
broccoli, fresh or frozen, 1 cup
* carrots
* celery
corn on the cob (5 inches long), fresh or frozen, 1 ear
* cranberry juice cocktail, low-calorie
* cucumber
* dates
* dill pickle spears (6 inches long)
* eggplant, 1 pound
* green beans, French-style, fresh or frozen, 1 cup
* green onion, 1
* green peas, early, frozen
green pepper, medium (3-inch diameter), 1
lettuce, 1 large head
lemon, fresh, 1 large
calories per tablespoon)
dry white wine, 1/2 cup
egg substitute, frozen
* molasses
* semi-condensed cream of mushroom soup, 7 1/2 ounces
low-sodium soy sauce
sour-cream and butter-flavor sprinkles
* mushrooms, canned (2 1/2 ounces)

* mushrooms, fresh, 10
onion, white, 1 medium
canned peaches, juice-packed, 1 1/2 cups
* canned pineapple slices, juice-packed, 1
canned pineapple crushed, juice-packed, 4 ounces
canned pineapple chunks, juice-packed, 8 ounces
potato, small (2 1/2-inch diameter, 4 1/2 ounces), 1
radish, 2
* salsa, canned in jars, 1
sweet red pepper, medium (3-inch diameter)
* strawberries (fresh or frozen without sugar), 1 cup
* tomatoe, medium (3-inch diameter), 1
* canned stewed tomatoes, Italian-style (with basil, garlic, and oregano), 12 1/2 ounces
* vegetable juice cocktail
zucchini, 1/4 cup

MISCELLANEOUS

all-purpose flour, 1/2 tablespoon
baking powder
* black bean soup, 16-ounce can
brown sugar
* catsup, 1 1/2 teaspoons
cider vinegar, 1 tablespoon
cornstarch
diet Italian dressing (6

WEEKS 5 AND 6
•••

HAVE ON HAND: STAPLES

* non-caloric beverages (water, coffee, tea, diet soft drinks)
* reduced-calorie bread (40 calories per slice)
* cereal (110 calories per ounce), choose from:
  Nabisco Shredded Wheat
  Kellogg's Frosted Mini-Wheats
  Kellogg's NutriGrain Wheat or Corn
  Oatmeal (not individual packages)
  Post Grape Nuts
  Ralston Purina Almond Delight
  Ralston Purina Sun Flakes Crispy Wheat & Rice
* Nature Valley Granola Bars (Almond, Cinnamon, or Oats 'n Honey)
* graham crackers
  low-calorie margarine (50 calories per tablespoon)
  low-calorie mayonnaise (40 calories per tablespoon)
  Parmesan cheese
  raisins
  salt
* saltine crackers
  skim milk
  vegetable cooking spray (butter flavor)
* vegetable cooking oil

HERBS, SPICES, SEASONINGS

  dried basil
* celery seed

  cinnamon
* cinnamon sticks
* whole cloves
* garlic cloves, 4
  garlic powder
  garlic salt (optional)
* ground ginger
* green chili peppers, chopped (4-ounce can)
* hot-pepper sauce
* ground lemon peel
* ground orange peel
* ground nutmeg
  paprika
* dried parsley
  dried thyme
  vanilla
  Worcestershire sauce

MEAT, FISH, POULTRY

  chicken breast halves (raw weight 4 ounces each), 3
* canned white meat chicken (2-ounce serving)
  imitation crab meat, 2 ounces
* eggs
* peanuts, dry-roasted, 4 1/2 ounces
  ground turkey, 1 pound
* canned turkey, white meat (2-ounce serving)
* canned tuna, water-packed (2-ounce serving)

FROZEN DINNERS

  Le Menu Light Style:
  3-Cheese Stuffed Shells, 1

Weight Watchers: Deluxe
Combination Pizza, 1
Stouffer's Right Course
Shrimp Primavera, 1
* Booth: Shrimp New
Orleans, 1
* Weight Watchers: Broccoli &
Cheese Baked Potato
* Lean Cuisine: Filet of Fish
Jardiniere with Souffléed
Potato

DAIRY PRODUCTS

* reduced-calorie sharp
cheddar cheese (50
calories/slice)
* cottage cheese, 1% fat
* ice milk, any flavor (100
calories per 1/2-cup serving)
* part-skim mozzarella cheese,
4 ounces
* plain yogurt, non-fat, 8
ounces
* fruited yogurt, non-fat,
sweetened with aspartame
(100 calories per 8 ounces)

BREADS, CEREALS

* 100% whole bran cereal
* corn tortillas
dried bread crumbs, 2
tablespoons
flour tortilla, (6-inch
diameter), 1
* macaroni (corkscrew or
plain)
* cinnamon-raisin English
muffin
* raisin bran cereal, 2 cups
white rice

* reduced-calorie Italian bread,
40 calories/slice, 8 slices
* reduced-calorie oatmeal
bread, 40 calories/slice
* oat bran waffles (frozen),
120 calories/waffle
* whole wheat pita bread
(4-inch diameter)

FRUITS, VEGETABLES, JUICES

* apple, medium (3-inch
diameter)
applesauce, unsweetened,
1 cup
bananas, medium (8 3/4
inches long), 4
* banana, ripe, large (9 3/4
inches long), 1
broccoli, fresh or frozen,
1 cup
* carrots
* celery
corn on the cob (5 inches
long), fresh or frozen, 1 ear
* cranberry juice cocktail,
low-calorie
* cucumber
* dates
* dill pickle spears (6 inches
long)
* eggplant, 1 pound
* grapefruit, small (3 3/4-inch
diameter)
* green onion, 1
* green peas, early, frozen
green pepper, medium
(3-inch diameter), 1
lettuce, 1 large head
lemon, fresh, 1 large
* mushrooms, canned (2 1/2
ounces)

* mushrooms, fresh, 10
  onion, white, 1 medium
* pears, fresh or canned,
  juice-packed
  canned pineapple slices,
  juice-packed, 1
  canned pineapple crushed,
  juice-packed, 4 ounces
  canned pineapple chunks,
  juice-packed, 8 ounces
  potato, small (2 1/2-inch
  diameter, 4 1/2 ounces), 1
  radish, 2
* salsa, canned in jars, 1
* spinach leaves, fresh
  sweet red pepper, medium
  (3-inch diameter), 1
* strawberries (fresh or frozen
  without sugar), 1 cup
* tomatoe, medium (3-inch
  diameter), 1
* canned stewed tomatoes,
  Italian-style (with basil,
  garlic, and oregano), 14 1/2
  ounces
* vegetable juice cocktail
  zucchini, 1/4 cup

diet Italian dressing (6
  calories per tablespoon)
dry white wine, 1/2 cup
egg substitute, frozen
* gelatin, sugar-free,
  strawberry (1 8-serving size
  or 2 4-serving size)
* molasses
* semi-condensed cream of
  mushroom soup, 7 1/2
  ounces
low-sodium soy sauce
sour-cream and butter-flavor
  sprinkles
* low-calorie sweetener

MISCELLANEOUS

all-purpose flour, 1/2
  tablespoon
* bacon bits, real
  baking powder
* black bean soup, 16-ounce
  can
  brown sugar
* catsup, 1 1/2 teaspoons
  cider vinegar, 1 tablespoon
* club soda, 1 cup
  cornstarch

21

Adapting the Diet for the Petite Woman

$\vdots$

Ninety-five percent of the women who have been on the recommended 1,400-1,300-1,200 calorie diet lose fat efficiently. There are a few women, however, who do not make progress. These women are usually shorter than 5 feet 2 inches and weigh 120 pounds or less.

If you fall into this category, lowering the weekly calories to 10, 1,100, and 1,000 works well. The following conversion table makes it easy for you to adapt the menus to 1,200 calories for weeks 1 and 2, 1,100 calories for weeks 3 and 4, and 1,000 calories for the final two weeks.

Do *not* use this conversion table unless you are shorter than 5 feet 2 inches tall and weigh 120 pounds or less. If you fall above this range you will *not* get faster results by consuming fewer calories. In fact, your results will be decreased because your energy to exercise will be reduced. Furthermore, the synergistic effect will not be as great. Regardless of your height and weight, the exercise program should remain unchanged.

HIP AND THIGH DIET CONVERSION
•••
(1200, 1100, 1000 Calories)

1. Breakfast =   no change necessary

2. Mid-morning Snack = omit

3. Lunch =   no change necessary

4. Afternoon Snack:
    Weeks 1–4 =   50 calories
    Weeks 5–6 =   (select 50-calorie snack for *either*
                            afternoon or evening snack, based on
                            hunger-problem time)

5. Dinner =   see specific daily changes below

6. Evening Snack:
    Weeks 1–2 =   no change necessary
    Weeks 3–4 =   100 calories (original snacks weeks
                            5–6)
    Weeks 5–6 =   (select 50-calorie snack for *either*
                            afternoon or evening snack, based on
                            hunger)

REVISED CALORIES:	Meal Total	Daily Total By Week
Monday Dinner omit: garlic bread add: ½ teaspoon vegetable oil to salad dressing	(352 calories)	(1204, 1104, 1004)
Tuesday Dinner have *only* 25 calories in fruit at dinner	(353 calories)	(1205, 1105, 1005)
Wednesday Dinner omit: graham crackers	(356 calories)	(1208, 1108, 1008)
Thursday Dinner omit: bread serve margarine over steamed broccoli	(350 calories)	(1202, 1102, 1002)

Friday Dinner omit: applesauce	(350 calories)	(1202, 1102, 1002)
Saturday Dinner omit: 1 meatball	(355 Calories)	(1207, 1107, 1007)
Sunday Dinner omit: granola reduce: green bean serving ½ cup	(355 calories)	(1205, 1105, 1005)

OPTIONAL MEALS

Weeks 3 & 4:

Monday Dinner Option omit: dates	(355 calories)
Thursday Dinner Option omit: dinner salad and dressing add: fruit salad from **Wednesday Dinner** (Wks. 1–6)	(357 calories)
Saturday Dinner Option omit: bread	(362 calories)

Weeks 5 & 6:

Wednesday Dinner Option omit: English muffin add: 1 tablespoon Home Granola	(350 calories)
Friday Dinner Option omit: graham cracker	(356 calories)
Sunday Dinner Option omit: ½ banana	(354 calories)

···**22**···
Holiday
Dieting Help

⋮

The first group of women who went through the Hot Hips and Fabulous Thighs program, as I mentioned in Chapter 1, did so during November and December. Perhaps the biggest deterrent to successful dieting at this time is the holiday pigout. Thanksgiving and Christmas feasting make a low-calorie eating plan difficult to follow.

To help combat this situation, I asked Brenda Hutchins—who did an excellent job on the menus and recipes for this book—to provide November and December dieters with some special holiday help. If you can get a handle on your eating during Thanksgiving and Christmas, you can surely transfer the mechanics to other festive times.

··● THANKSGIVING DAY

Prepare for the Thanksgiving meal by eliminating the juice from breakfast, the fruit from lunch, and changing the snacks as directed. This will conserve approximately 282 calories.

Do *not* try to cut calories by omitting several meals prior to the Thanksgiving feast. You will succeed at only one thing: sounding your body's famine alarm. In response to this signal, the body tends to conserve fat. Your scheme will backfire, causing your body to hoard more calories. It will not give you the extra caloric buffer for gorging that you imagined.

With the suggestions below you'll be able to get through Thanksgiving with both enjoyment and minimal damage to the progress you've made so far. You'll also be a veteran when it comes to Christmas preparations.

Total calories: 1,298

- **Breakfast:** 220 calories (OMIT JUICE)
  - Basic Breakfast One
    or
  - Basic Breakfast Two
  - Basic Breakfast Three
    or
  - Basic Breakfast Four

- **Mid-morning Snack:** 50 calories (USE THIS SNACK INSTEAD)
  1 serving fruit (50)
    or
  ¹/₂ cup fruited, non-fat yogurt (50)

- **Lunch:** 302 calories (OMIT FRUIT)
  - Basic Lunch One
    or
  - Basic Lunch Two
  - Basic Lunch Three
    or
  - Basic Lunch Four

- **Mid-afternoon Fruit Snack:** 50 calories
  - 1 serving fruit (50)
    or
  - ¹/₂ cup fruited, non-fat yogurt (50)

- **Dinner:** 676 calories
  4 slices turkey, light meat without skin, (2 ¹/₂ inches × 1 ⁵/₈ inches × ¹/₄ inches thick, 3 ounces, preferably not pre-basted) (150)
  ¹/₂ cup dressing (170)
  ¹/₄ cup Defatted Gravy, Recipe #19 (25)
- *CHOICE OF ONE:* (68)
  ¹/₂ cup diced potatoes, boiled and mashed with 1 ¹/₂ tablespoons plain non-fat yogurt
  OR
  ¹/₄ cup vacuum-packed sweet potatoes heated with ¹/₂ teaspoon low-calorie margarine
  Sprinkle of cinnamon
  Plus:
  1 cup French-style green beans, steamed (31)
  2 tablespoons Cranberry Sauce, Recipe #20 (17)
  ¹/₂ cup Congealed Strawberry Salad, Recipe #21 (18)
  1 slice pumpkin pie (¹/₆ of 10-ounce Banquet) (197)
  Noncaloric beverage

••• CHRISTMAS DAY

Here is a similar strategy you may use for Christmas day. Compared to Thanksgiving, the Christmas calories are slightly higher.

Total calories: 1400

- **Breakfast:**   220 calories (OMIT JUICE)
  - Basic Breakfast One
    or
  - Basic Breakfast Two
  - Basic Breakfast Three
    or
  - Basic Breakfast Four

- **Mid-morning Snack:**   50 calories
    (USE THIS SNACK INSTEAD)
- 1 serving fruit (50)
    or
- ½ cup fruited, non-fat yogurt (50)

- **Lunch:**   302 calories (OMIT FRUIT)
  - Basic Lunch One
    or
  - Basic Lunch Two
  - Basic Lunch Three
    or
  - Basic Lunch Four

- **Mid-afternoon Fruit Snack:**   50 calories
  - 1 serving fruit (50)
    or
  - ½ cup fruited, non-fat yogurt (50)

- **Dinner:**   778 calories
  Holiday Nog, Recipe #22 (159)
  Layered Salad, Recipe #23 (80)
  Sweet Potato Treasure, Recipe #24 (97)
  Christmas Ham with Citrus Glaze, Recipe #25 (160)
  2 tablespoons Cran-Raspberry Sauce, Recipe #26 (10)
  1 brown-and-serve roll (85)
  1 teaspoon diet margarine (17)
  Apple-Almond Bar, Recipe #27 (70)
  ½ cup ice milk (100)
  Noncaloric beverage

● *Recipe #19*

DEFATTED GRAVY
● ● ●

STEP 1: DEFAT DRIPPINGS

The *easy way* is to quick-chill pan drippings in a cup in the freezer until the fat rises to the surface and hardens. Lift fat off and discard.

Rush method: Pour hot drippings into a tall, narrow heat-proof container and wait two minutes, or until the fat reaches the surface. Extract fat with a bulb-type baster.

Canned broth: Canned broth can be used in place of meat drippings. Open can and remove any fat globules on the surface.

STEP 2: MEASURE

Measure stock and heat to boiling. For each cup of stock, combine in a SEPARATE CUP:

2 tablespoons flour
¼ cup water

Stir until smooth and lump-free. (*NEVER* add flour directly to a hot liquid; it will lump.) Stir flour mixture into simmering stock broth until thickened. If it gets too thick, thin it by adding a little water gradually.

STEP 3: SEASON

Season gravy to your taste: salt, pepper, onion powder, or herbs.

STEP 4: MEASURE

Now you have successfully created low-fat gravy, don't get carried away. Remember to *measure* your portion-size carefully.

Calories: 25 per ¼ cup

• *Recipe #20*

CRANBERRY SAUCE
— • • • —

 2 cups fresh or frozen (thawed) cranberries
 1 cup water
 3 teaspoons cornstarch
18 packets low-calorie sweetener

Combine cranberries and 1/2 cup water in a heavy
saucepan. Bring to a boil. Cover; reduce heat and
simmer until berries have popped (about 5 minutes).
Dissolve cornstarch in remaining water. Add to
cranberries and continue to cook, stirring constantly,
until syrup thickens. Remove from heat and cool
slightly; stir in sweetener. Serve warm or chilled.

Yield: 1 1/2 cups
Calories: 17 per two-tablespoon serving

• *Recipe #21*

CONGEALED STRAWBERRY SALAD
— • • • —

 1   package (8-serving size) or 2 (4-serving size)
          sugar-free strawberry-flavored gelatin
1 1/2 cups boiling water
 1/2   teaspoon ground ginger
 1   cup club soda
 8   ice cubes
1 1/2 cups strawberries, sliced
 9   lettuce leaves

Sprinkle gelatin into a 13-inch × 9-inch casserole dish;
add boiling water and stir until completely dissolved.
Add ginger, club soda, and ice; stir until ice is melted
and mixture is slightly thickened. Mix in strawberries.
Chill until set, about one hour. Slice into 9 equal
servings and serve on lettuce leaf.

Yield: 9 servings
Calories: 18 per serving

● *Recipe #22*

HOLIDAY NOG
— ● ● ● —

3   cups low-fat milk
1   cup evaporated skim milk
1   cup light rum
    OR
4   teaspoons rum flavoring
½   cup frozen egg substitute (thawed)
2   packets low-calorie sweetener
1   teaspoon vanilla extract
    Nutmeg

Combine all ingredients, except nutmeg, in a blender or food processor. Cover and process on low speed about 30 seconds, or until frothy. Pour into cups and sprinkle with nutmeg. Serve at once.

Yield: 8 servings (¾ cup)
Calories: 159 per serving

● *Recipe #23*

LAYERED SALAD
— ● ● ● —

1   10-ounce bag frozen sweet peas, thawed
1   cup cherry tomatoes (8 tomatoes, about 5.3
    ounces)
½   cup plain non-fat yogurt
6   tablespoons reduced-calorie mayonnaise or salad
    dressing
1   tablespoon skim milk
¾   teaspoon dried sweet basil
6   cups torn lettuce
1   cup sliced fresh mushrooms
½   cup shredded carrots
½   cup Bermuda onion rings, very thinly sliced
½   cup cheese croutons

Place frozen peas in a colander. Run hot water over them just until thawed. Drain well. Meanwhile, cut tomatoes into quarters and place in a covered container, then chill.

Combine yogurt, mayonnaise or salad dressing, skim milk, and basil (crush just before adding) in a small mixing bowl. Set dressing aside.

Assemble salad: Select a large salad bowl (preferably clear glass). Arrange layers of lettuce, mushrooms, peas, carrots, onion rings; spread dressing over top. Cover and chill for 2 to 3 hours. Before serving, top with tomatoes and croutons.

Yield: 8 servings
Calories: 80 per serving

• *Recipe #24*

SWEET POTATO TREASURE
— • • • —

1   18-ounce can sweet potatoes, drained
1   8 1/4-ounce can juice-packed, crushed pineapple, drained (reserve juice)
1   egg
2   tablespoons diet margarine
1/2 teaspoon salt
    Dash pepper
1/4 teaspoon ground nutmeg
    Butter-flavor cooking spray

Preheat oven to 375 degrees. Mash sweet potatoes and set aside. Combine remaining ingredients (except spray) in a medium-sized mixing bowl; mix well. Whip sweet potatoes together with pineapple mixture. Treat eight custard dishes or casserole with cooking spray. Spoon even amounts of sweet potato mixture into dishes. Bake at 375 degrees for 35–40 minutes. Allow to set for 5 minutes before serving.

Yield: 8 servings
Calories: 97 per serving

- *Recipe #25*

CHRISTMAS HAM WITH CITRUS GLAZE
—————— • • • ——————

Choose a 3- to 5-pound pre-cooked canned ham (such as Hormel Black Label boneless, skinless) trimmed of all separable fat. Reheat ham according to package directions. During last half hour, pour half of Citrus Glaze over ham. Use pastry brush to coat evenly. Continue baking at 350 degrees for 30 minutes or until glazed. Serve remaining sauce with ham.

Yield: 8 servings (4 ounces ham with 2 tablespoons glaze)
Calories: 160 per serving

Citrus Glaze:

¼   cup Brown SugarTwin
2   tablespoons cornstarch
⅛   teaspoon salt
1   cup unsweetened orange juice
    Reserved unsweetened pineapple juice, from Recipe #24 (add enough water to equal 1 cup)
¼   teaspoon ground cinnamon
⅛   teaspoon ground cloves

Mix Brown SugarTwin, cornstarch, and salt together in a saucepan. Add orange juice, pineapple juice, and spices. Cook over medium heat until mixture thickens, stirring constantly. Remove from heat. Pour half of sauce over ham. Use pastry brush to coat ham evenly.

"The Thanksgiving and Christmas menus and recipes helped me make it through the holidays without gaining an ounce. In fact, I lost a pound."

JOCELYN BENBOW
— •●• —

age: 19
height: 5'7"

LOST 9 ½ pounds of fat, **RESHAPED** her body by adding 1 pound of muscle, and **TRIMMED** 3 inches off her waist, 1 ⅞ inches off her hips, and 1 inch off her upper thighs in six weeks.

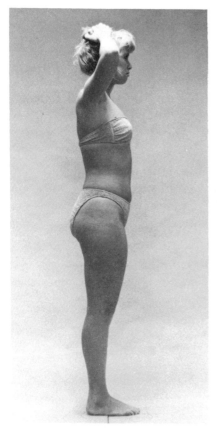
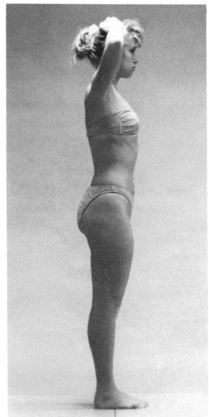

Before   **After**

- *Recipe #26*

CRAN-RASPBERRY SAUCE
—— •••——

1   4-serving-size sugar-free raspberry gelatin
¼   cup water
1   cup low-calorie cranberry juice cocktail
¾   cup unsweetened applesauce

Dissolve gelatin in ¼ cup boiling water. Add cranberry juice cocktail and applesauce; mix well. Chill until firm.

Yield: 8 servings (2 tablespoons per serving)
Calories: 10 calories per serving

- *Recipe #27*

APPLE-ALMOND BAR
—— •••——

½   cup all-purpose flour
½   cup sugar
1   teaspoon baking powder
1   teaspoon ground cinnamon
¼   teaspoon salt
¼   cup frozen egg substitute (thawed)
1   teaspoon vanilla extract
1   cup chopped apple
¼   cup slivered almonds
    Butter-flavor cooking spray
¼   cup sifted powdered sugar
2   teaspoons hot water
⅛   teaspoon almond-flavored extract

Preheat oven to 400 degrees. Combine first 5 ingredients in a large bowl; stir well. Add egg substitute and vanilla; stir until well blended. Mix in chopped apple and slivered almonds.

Treat an 8-inch square baking pan with cooking spray. Spoon batter into baking pan and bake at 400 degrees for 15 to 20 minutes or until a wooden pick inserted in center comes out clean. Remove pan from oven and allow to cool on a wire rack.

Combine powdered sugar, hot water, and almond extract; stir until smooth. Drizzle glaze over top and cut into 2-inch square bars.

Yield: 16 bars   **Calories:** 70 per bar

••• SHOPPING LIST

This shopping list includes only the items required for Christmas dinner preparation.

HERBS, SPICES, SEASONINGS

almond extract
dried basil
ground cinnamon
ground cloves
ground nutmeg
• rum flavoring (if not using liquor in Holiday Nog)
vanilla

MEAT, FISH, POULTRY

eggs, 1
frozen egg substitute, 3/4 cup
canned ham, 3 pounds (such as Hormel: Black Label)

DAIRY PRODUCTS

evaporated skim milk, 1 cup
low-fat milk, 3 cups
plain yogurt, non-fat, 1/2 cup

FRUITS, VEGETABLES, JUICES

apple, 1 cup chopped
applesauce, unsweetened, 3/4 cup
carrots, 1/2 cup shredded
cranberry juice cocktail, low-calorie, 1 cup

green peas, sweet, frozen, 10-ounce bag
lettuce, 1 large head
mushrooms, fresh, 1 cup sliced
onion, Bermuda, 1 medium
unsweetened orange juice, 1 cup
canned pineapple crushed, juice-packed, 8 1/4 ounces
canned sweet potatoes, 18 ounces
cherry tomatoes, 8 (about 5.3 ounces)

MISCELLANEOUS

all-purpose flour, 1/2 cup
almonds, slivered, 1/4 cup
baking powder
Brown SugarTwin, 1/4 cup
cornstarch
gelatin, sugar-free, raspberry (1 4-serving size)
reduced-calorie mayonnaise, 6 tablespoons
light rum
powdered sugar
sugar, 1/2 cup
low-calorie sweetener

···23···

Hip and Thigh Freehand Exercise Routines

⋮

The dictionary defines exercise as ". . . exertion of the muscles to maintain bodily health."

Exercise is better defined as "movement against resistance." Without resistance, there is no effective exercise.

For your body to become more shapely and leaner, your muscles have to become larger and stronger. Muscles don't become larger and stronger unless they are taxed with a progressive overload. Once they are overloaded, a chemical reaction takes place within the body that causes your muscles to become larger, stronger, and shapelier.

The quality of the overload or resistance determines the value of the exercise. That's the major problem with freehand exercises or calisthenics. It's difficult to overload your body by using the weight of your own arms, legs, or torso. At least it is if you exercised in the traditional style using fast, jerky movements.

This has changed with the application of super-slow repetitions and sustained contractions.

··· SUPER-SLOW SUSTAINED CONTRACTIONS

Most super-slow repetitions require you to lift your body weight or body part slowly to the top position, where the sustained contraction usually occurs. Sustained contractions mean you intensely squeeze the involved muscles for an extended time. Most exercisers bounce in and out of the top position. In super-slow sustained contractions you do just the opposite.

Hold the contracted position for at least 10 seconds. Gradually within the next six weeks, by adding 2 or 3 seconds per workout, try to work up to a 30-second hold. Return smoothly back to the starting position and repeat. Each exercise is continued for 5 repetitions, which takes from 75 to 180 seconds per set.

Once you can do more than three minutes of any exercise, the efficiency of muscle stimulations drops. There's no need to continue any freehand exercise longer than three minutes.

With super-slow sustained contractions, it should be obvious that your breathing is important. Your breathing should be emphasized in a specific way for best results.

••• HOW TO BREATHE

First, do not hold your breath during the exercises. Doing so can cause your blood pressure to elevate to high levels. Keep your mouth open and breathe, especially during the last part of the exercise.

Second, take short rapid breaths with emphasis on blowing out rather than taking in large gulps of air. Try to ventilate just enough so your breathing never stops.

Many of the women who have learned the technique note that the method of breathing is like that taught in Lamaze childbirth classes. That's true. Both stress that when the work gets tough, relax your face, and breathe—breathe—breathe.

••• WARMING UP AND COOLING DOWN

Before exercising it's a good idea to take several minutes to loosen up. Do a few easy movements, such as bringing one knee to your chest and then the other, torso rotations, and swinging your arms in slow circles. After your workout, cool down by walking around the exercise area and getting a drink of cold water. Continue to move until your elevated heart rate subsides.

••• THE FREEHAND ROUTINES

The super-slow freehand routines center around three nonconsecutive-day, 30-minute workouts per week. You do nine exercises for Weeks 1 and 2, ten exercises for the middle two weeks, and eleven for Weeks 5 and 6.

With the workouts, you'll be amazed at what's happening to the tightness and shape of your hips and thighs. In six weeks you'll see significant changes.

The following routines can all be done with rhythmic music in the background. In fact, several large fitness clubs in Dallas offered supervised classes with approximately 15 women per group. An instructor with a stop watch called out guidelines as she led the women through each exercise. Most agreed that the background music was helpful.

WEEKS 1 & 2

1. Wide squat against wall
2. Hip raise
3. Inner thigh lift
4. Reverse leg raise
5. Trunk curl
6. Donkey kick
7. Negative push-up
8. Hip raise
9. Wide squat against wall

WEEKS 3 & 4

1. Wide squat against wall
2. Hip raise
3. Narrow squat against wall
4. Inner thigh lift
5. Reverse leg raise
6. Trunk curl
7. Donkey kick
8. Negative push-up
9. Hip raise
10. Wide squat against wall

WEEKS 5 & 6

1. Wide squat against wall
2. Hip raise
3. Narrow squat against wall
4. Inner thigh lift
5. Reverse leg raise
6. Trunk curl
7. Donkey kick
8. Negative push-up
9. Narrow squat against wall
10. Hip raise
11. Wide squat against wall

Wide squat against wall (for thighs and buttocks): Stand erect and lean back against a smooth, sturdy wall. Place heels six inches wider apart than shoulders and one-and-one-half to two feet away from wall. Adjust hands on hips. Put a pillow at bottom of wall. Bend at hips and knees and slide down wall until tops of thighs are parallel to floor. Hold for 10 seconds. Push back to top position and immediately lower back to parallel position. Do not lock knees in top position. Keep them bent slightly. Repeat for 5 sustained-contraction repetitions.

Increase the duration of each repetition by several seconds each workout. Your goal is to do 5 30-second repetitions. The entire set should take no longer than three minutes.

Note: You'll do a second set of the wide squat at the end of each workout.

Hip raise (for buttocks): Lie on your back on floor. Slide feet under knees. Raise hips upward. Keep head, shoulders, and hands on floor. Arch lower back slightly. Contract buttocks intensely and hold for 10 seconds. Lower hips back to floor, but do not rest. Repeat for 5 sustained-contraction repetitions.

Increase the duration of each repetition by several seconds each workout. Your goal is to do 5 30-second repetitions. The entire set should take no longer than three minutes.

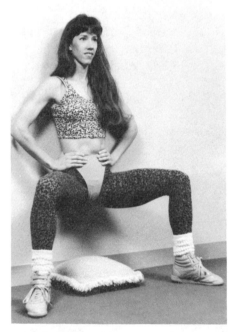

Wide Squat: Bottom position.

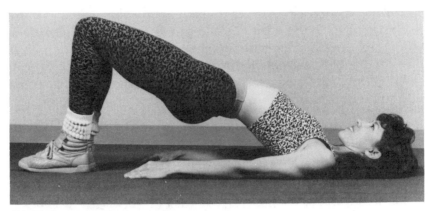

Hip Raise: Contracted position.

After hip raise, release tension in your back and hips by curling up into a ball for 5 seconds.

Note: You'll do a second set of the hip raise at the end of each workout.

Narrow squat against wall (for buttocks and thighs): Do the narrow squat in a similar manner to the wide squat with one exception. Place feet only two inches apart. Also, progress in same fashion as the wide squat.

Note: You'll do a second set of the narrow squat during Weeks 5 and 6.

Narrow Squat: Bottom position.

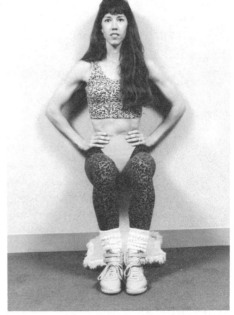

Inner thigh lift (for inner thighs): Lie on your side and stabilize your torso. Bend top knee and put foot on floor in front of other thigh. Grasp ankle with top hand. Raise bottom leg as high as possible. Hold in sustained contraction for 10 seconds. Lower to floor. Repeat for 5 sustained-contraction repetitions. Lie on other side and repeat for opposite thigh.

Increase the duration of each repetition by several seconds each workout. Your goal is to do 5 30-second repetitions. This entire set should take no longer than three minutes.

Reverse leg raise (for buttocks): Lie face down on floor. Place hands palms-down by hips. Lift both legs backward as high as possible. Hold in top position and squeeze buttocks together intensely for 10 seconds. Lower thighs to floor. Repeat for 5 sustained-contraction repetitions.

Increase the duration of each repetition by several seconds each workout. Your goal is to do 5 30-second repetitions. The entire set should take no longer than three minutes.

After reverse leg raise, roll over on your back. Release tension in your back and hips by curling up into a ball for 5 seconds.

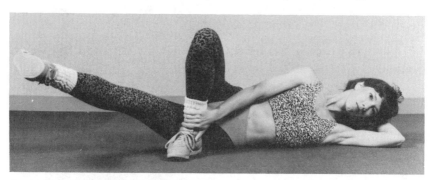

Inner Thigh Lift: Contracted position.

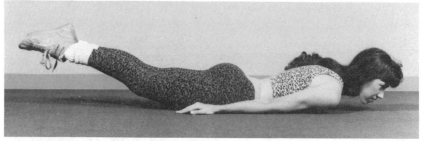

Reverse Leg Raise: Contracted position.

Trunk Curl: Contracted position.

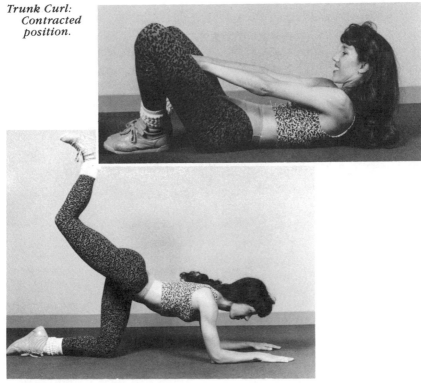

Donkey Kick: Contracted position.

Trunk curl (for midsection): Lie face up on floor. Bring heels close to buttocks and spread knees. Interlace hands and place over midsection. Curl shoulders gradually off floor and reach with hands between thighs. Only one-third of a standard sit-up can be performed. Pause in the top position for 10 seconds and keep reaching. Lower shoulders to floor. Repeat for 5 sustained-contraction repetitions.

Increase the duration of each repetition by several seconds each workout. Your goal is to do 5 30-second repetitions. The entire set should take you no longer than three minutes.

Donkey kick (for buttocks): Kneel on hands and knees. Pull one knee to chest and smoothly extend it high above and beyond the back. Pause in top position for 10 seconds. Try to put bottom of foot on ceiling. Lower knee to chest. Repeat for 5 sustained-contraction repetitions. Switch knees and repeat for other leg.

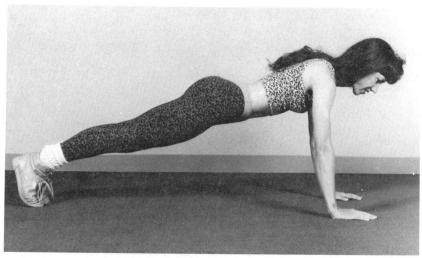

Negative Push-Up: Starting position.

Increase the duration of each repetition by several seconds each workout. Your goal is to do 5 30-second repetitions. This entire set should take no longer than three minutes.

After the donkey kick, roll over on your back. Release tension in your back and hips by curling up into a ball for 5 seconds.

Negative push-up (for upper body): This is the only upper body exercise you'll do and the only one you'll do in a negative, or lowering-only, manner. Assume a standard push-up position on toes and hands with body stiff. Lower body to floor by bending arms slowly in 10 seconds. Do not try to push yourself up to top position. When you reach floor, bend knees, straighten arms, get back on toes, and stiffen body once again. Repeat 5 times.

Add repetitions, instead of time, to this exercise. Your goal is to do 10 10-second negative repetitions.

···24···
Hip and Thigh Nautilus Routines

You've probably heard of Nautilus equipment. Or perhaps you've exercised on it.

Nautilus is the most popular of the exercise machines that are sold in the United States. Most of them are found in fitness centers, YMCAs, and health clubs. If you have access to Nautilus, use it according to the instructions provided in this chapter. If you do not have Nautilus available, but have another type of equipment, you may be able to use it instead. Check with the management to be sure the equipment applies.

Approximately half of the women who were supervised through the Hot Hips and Fabulous Thighs program exercised on Nautilus equipment. The other half employed freehand exercises. Both forms of exercise yielded outstanding results. When the muscle increases were compared, however, the Nautilus-trained women produced 33 percent better gains. Nautilus provides a more systematic way of progressing the overload or resistance.

··· WORK BETWEEN 4 AND 8 REPETITIONS

Your guideline number of super-slow repetitions is 4 to 8. If you cannot do at least 4 repetitions, the weight on the machine is too heavy. If you can do 8 or more, the weight is too light.

Important: If you can do another repetition, never stop an exercise, regardless of the number. Perform as many repetitions as possible in good form, and then try one more. When upward movement becomes impossible, continue to sustain the contraction for another 5 seconds or so.

When you can do 8 or more super-slow repetitions on any Nautilus exercise, increase the weight by approximately 5 percent at your next workout. This should reduce your repetitions to 4 or 5. Strive to work up to 8 or more repetitions during the following few training sessions. With each workout you should progress in resistance or repetitions.

••• NAUTILUS ROUTINES

Apply the following Nautilus routines for lasting results.

WEEKS 1 & 2	WEEKS 3 & 4	WEEKS 5 & 6
1. Leg Curl	1. Leg Curl	1. Leg Curl
2. Leg Extension	2. Leg Extension	2. Leg Extension
3. Leg Press	3. Leg Press	3. Leg Press
4. Hip Abduction	4. Hip Abduction	4. Hip Abduction
5. Hip Adduction	5. Hip Adduction	5. Hip Adduction
6. Pullover	6. Pullover	6. Pullover
7. Bench Press	7. Bench Press	7. Bench Press
8. Abdominal	8. Abdominal	8. Abdominal
	9. Leg Press	9. Leg Press
		10. Hip Abduction

Leg Curl (for back thighs): Lie face down on machine. Place back ankles under roller pads with knees just over edge of bench. Grasp handles to keep body from moving. Curl both legs in 10 seconds and try to touch heels to buttocks. Pause. Lower in 5 seconds. Repeat for maximum repetitions.

Leg Extension (for front thighs): Sit in machine. Lean forward and place shins behind roller pads. Adjust seat back to buttocks. Make sure knees are aligned with axis of rotation of movement arm. Axis is marked with a red dot. Fasten seat belt. Straighten both legs slowly in 10 seconds. Pause. Lower legs in 5 seconds. Repeat for maximum repetitions.

Leg Press (for buttocks and thighs): Adjust seat back to comfortable position and note placement of pin. Adjust seat carriage until knees, with feet in proper position on movement arm, are near chest. The closer the seat is to the movement arm, the longer the range of motion and the harder the exercise. Note seat position

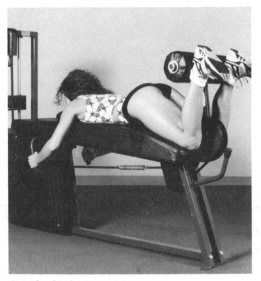

Leg Curl: Contracted position.

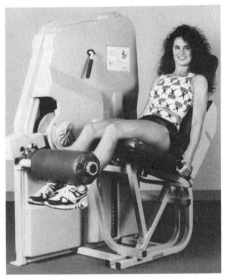

Leg Extension: Mid-range position.

by bottom handle of carriage. Both seat back and seat carriage should be adjusted to same position each time you do the exercise.

Sit in machine with feet placed evenly on foot pedal of movement arm. Grasp handles lightly by hips. Push with feet and straighten both legs slowly in 10 seconds. Do not lock knees. Keep them bent slightly. Lower weight in 5 seconds. Repeat for maximum repetitions.

Note: You'll do a second set of the Leg Press during Weeks 3–6.

Leg Press: Starting position.

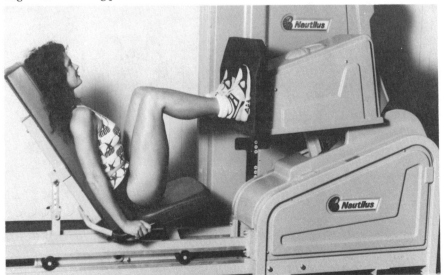

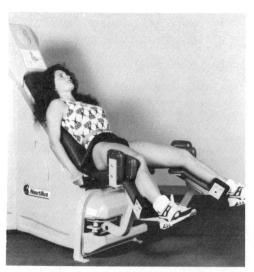

Hip Abduction: Contracted position.

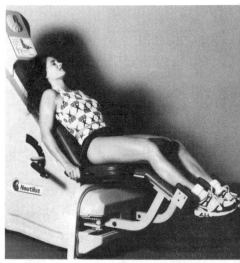

Hip Adduction: Contracted position.

**Bench Press:
Top position.**

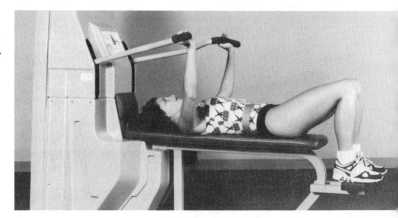

Pullover: Stretched position.

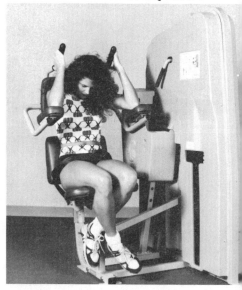

Abdominal: Contracted position.

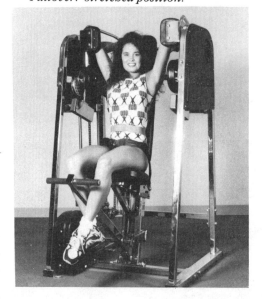

Hip Abduction (for outer hips): Sit in machine and place legs on movement arms. (Small women may require an extra back pad and additional thigh pads.) Fasten seat belt. Keep head and shoulders against seat back. Push knees and thighs apart to widest position slowly in 10 seconds. Pause. Return to knees-together position in 5 seconds. Repeat for maximum repetitions.

Note: You'll do a second set of the Hip Abduction during Weeks 5 and 6.

Hip Adduction (for inner thighs): Adjust lever on right side of machine for range of movement. Sit in machine and place knees and ankles on movement arms in a spread-legged position. (Small women may require an extra back pad.) Fasten seat belt. Keep head and shoulders against seat back. Pull knees and thighs together slowly in 10 seconds. Pause. Return to stretched position in 5 seconds. Repeat for maximum repetitions.

Pullover (for upper back): Adjust seat so shoulders are aligned with axes of rotation of movement arm. Axes are marked with red dots. Fasten seat belt. Leg press foot pedal until elbow pads approach chin level. Place elbows on pads and hands against curved portion of crossbar. Remove feet from pedal and rotate elbows back into comfortable stretch. This is starting position. Rotate elbows forward and down slowly in 10 seconds. Pause. Return to stretched position in 5 seconds. Repeat for maximum repetitions.

Bench Press (for chest, shoulders, and upper arms): Lie face up on bench with handles beside chest. Grasp handles lightly. Stabilize body by placing feet flat on floor, or on step at end of bench. Press handles upward slowly in 10 seconds. Lower the handles in 5 seconds. Repeat for maximum repetitions.

Abdominal (for midsection): Sit in machine. Adjust seat so navel aligns with red dot on side of machine. Fasten seat belt across hips. Pull knees together and cross ankles. Place elbows on pads and grasp handles lightly. Expand chest, pull gradually with elbows, and slowly shorten distance between rib cage and pelvis in 10 seconds. Pause. Return to starting position in 5 seconds. Repeat for maximum repetitions.

···*25*···
After Six Weeks: Making More Progress

Okay, so you've finished the program and still have some pounds and inches to lose. You can only lose a certain amount of fat per day, per week, and per six weeks. In fact, the most fat lost in six weeks by any of the 118 women who went through the program was 20 pounds.

If you had more than 20 pounds of fat that you needed to reduce, there's a high probability that it's going to take you longer than six weeks. If you're in this category, here's what to do next.

••• MAKE ANOTHER COMMITMENT

Decide now—right this minute—that you want to continue. You've already taken some major steps toward reaching your goal of Hot Hips and Fabulous Thighs. You've made significant progress by sticking with the plan for six weeks. Make a commitment for another six weeks, or less, if you believe you can reach your goal sooner.

Several women committed to the program four times, 24 weeks, before they reached their satisfaction level with their hips and thighs. Simply turn the week-by-week dieting and exercising into week-by-week steps which move you closer and closer to your ideal muscle/fat ratio.

••• TAKE A WEEK OFF

You may think I'm in contradiction if I tell you to take a week off after I just asked you to make a commitment to further dieting and exercising. Most of the women who continued with the program felt that a week off renewed their enthusiasm.

Be careful not to gorge yourself with food. You probably would have difficulty doing so even if you tried. Simply eat approximately 500 more calories per day than you were eating during Weeks 5 and 6. Keep drinking your water: at least 1 5/8 gallons a day, or thirteen 16-ounce bottles, as recommended in Chapter 15.

After a week off you'll be amazed at how eager you are to repeat the six-week course.

••• REPEAT THE DIET

Six weeks ago, in two-week phases, you gradually decreased your calories from 1,400 to 1,300 to 1,200 per day. Now that you've added a few extra pounds of muscle to your body, you should be able to go through the same descending-calorie plan with similar or even better results.

Furthermore, this time around you'll have more flexibility in the menus and recipes. With an understanding of the holiday ideas in Chapter 22 and the special weekend recipes in Chapter 27, and with a little planning, you'll be able to add substantial variety to the standard eating plan. Just be sure your daily calories remain at the appropriate level.

••• MODIFY THE EXERCISE

You should continue to perform your muscle-building exercise in the super-slow style three times per week. With the freehand exercises, however, it becomes increasingly difficult to make the movements harder. Soon your hips and thighs will become so strong that you'll be able to perform some of the exercises for longer than three minutes without fatiguing. When this happens you will *not* be stimulating your muscles to the maximum level. At this point the exercise must not be made *longer* but *harder*. Harder and more progressive exercise for the hips and thighs is best performed on Nautilus equipment.

"Last year after Christmas, I made a commitment to myself that I was going to get rid of this fat, and that I was going to get my hips and thighs into great shape.

"My progress was steady and after three times through the program I finally reached my goal. I did it, I did it, I did it! I feel terrific!"

LINDA NAGY
• • •

age: 36

height: 5'4"

LOST 22 pounds of fat, **RESHAPED** her body by adding 4 ½ pounds of muscle, and **TRIMMED** 4 ⅛ inches off her waist, 4 ⅜ inches off her hips, and 6 ⅛ inches off her upper thighs in eighteen weeks.

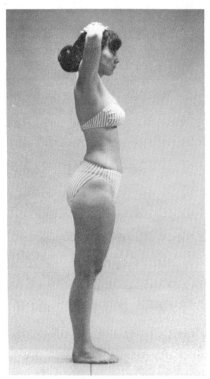 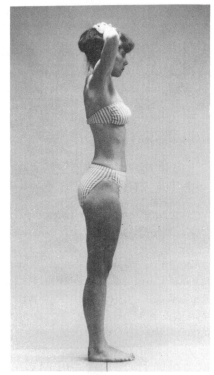

Before   **After**

When you can perform the majority of your freehand exercises for three minutes or longer, I suggest that you graduate to the Nautilus routines as detailed in Chapter 24. With the prescribed Nautilus routines you should continue to make progress for many months.

In either case, always strive to improve your muscle/fat ratio. Remember, it's your muscles that provide shape to your body, burn fat for energy, and raise your metabolic rate for sustained weight control.

••• ONE DAY AT A TIME

Patience is truly a virtue when it comes to losing those last few pounds and inches.

Hang in there. Those fat cells can shrink. Your dream, if it is realistic, can be accomplished. It does take time, however.

Be patient. Stick to the plan in this book. Make action your ally.

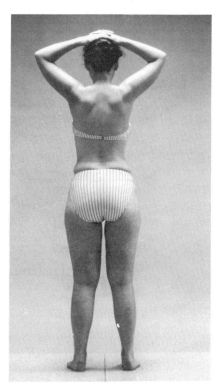 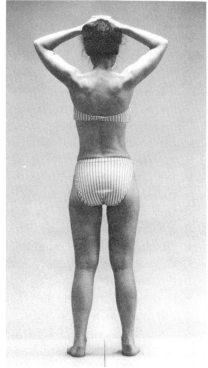

Before   **After**

···26···

After Six Weeks: Maintaining Your Weight

:

Once you reach your goal—whether it takes six weeks, twelve weeks, or more—a long-term maintenance program becomes of ultimate importance.

Your goal now is to maintain your ideal body weight, percent body fat, and hip and thigh size. The secrets to maintenance are in *the mechanics*—the mechanics of successful dieting and the mechanics of successful exercising.

••• APPLY THE MECHANICS

In summary form, here are the salient mechanics used so far:

- Focus on improving your muscle/fat ratio by building muscle and losing fat simultaneously.
- Descend your daily calories gradually from 1,400 to 1,300 to 1,200.
- Keep your daily calories balanced by consuming 50 percent carbohydrates, 30 percent fat, and 20 percent protein. The menus in this book are designed to do this for you.
- Drink from 16 to 26 glasses of cold water each day.
- Exercise progressively on three non-consecutive days per week.
- Move slower, never faster, if in doubt about the speed of movement on each repetition.
- Look for ways to make your exercise harder, not easier.
- Rest and relax on your non-exercise days.

150

MAINTENANCE GUIDELINES FOR CALORIES

Food	For 1,500 Calories	For 1,600 Calories	For 1,700 Calories	For 1,800 Calories	For 1,900 Calories	For 2,000 Calories	For 2,100 Calories	For 2,200 Calories	Notes
Meat Group	3 servings (or a total of 7 ounces cooked weight)	3 servings (or a total of 7 ounces cooked weight)	3 servings (or a total of 7 ounces cooked weight)	3½ servings (or a total of 9 ounces cooked weight)	4 servings (or a total of 10 ounces cooked weight)	4 servings (or a total of 10 ounces cooked weight)	4 servings (or a total of 10 ounces cooked weight)	4½ servings (or a total of 12 ounces cooked weight)	Choose lean, well-trimmed meats: beef, veal, lamb, pork. Poultry and fish should have skin removed. One egg can be substituted for 1 serving meat. One cup dried beans or peas can be substituted for 1 serving meat. One ounce lean meat = 60 calories.
Milk Group	2 cups whole milk	2 cups whole milk	2 cups whole milk, 1 cup fortified skim milk	2 cups whole milk, 1 cup fortified skim milk	2 cups whole milk, 1 cup fortified skim milk	2 cups whole milk, 2 cups fortified skim milk	2 cups whole milk, 2 cups fortified skim milk	2 cups whole milk, 2 cups fortified skim milk	Two cups milk mean two 8-ounce measuring cups. One cup low-fat plain yogurt may be substituted for 1 cup whole milk. One ounce hard or soft cheese may be substituted for 1 cup whole milk. One cup skim milk = 100 calories. One cup whole milk = 150 calories.
Fruits and Vegetables Group	4 servings	5 servings	5 servings	6 servings	6 servings	6 servings	6 servings	6 servings	One fruit serving = 1 medium fruit, 2 small fruits, ½ banana, ¼ cantaloupe, 10–12 grapes or cherries, 1 cup fresh berries, or ½ cup fresh, canned, or frozen unsweetened fruit juice. Include one citrus fruit or other good source of vitamin C daily. One fruit or vegetable serving = 50–75 calories. One vegetable serving = ½ cup cooked or 1 cup raw leafy vegetable. Include one dark or deep yellow vegetable or other good source of vitamin A at least every other day.
Breads and Cereals Group	5 servings	6 servings	6 servings	6 servings	6 servings	6 servings	7 servings	7 servings	One serving = 1 slice bread; 1 small dinner roll; ½ cup cooked cereal, noodles, macaroni, spaghetti, rice, or cornmeal; 1 ounce (about 1 cup) ready-to-eat unsweetened iron-fortified cereal. One bread or cereal serving = 75 calories.
Other Group	3 servings	3 servings	3 servings	3 servings	3 servings	3 servings	4 servings	4 servings	1 serving = 1 teaspoon butter, margarine, or oil; 6 nuts; 2 teaspoons salad dressing; or 35 calories or less of other fluid.

"***R**ecently, I visited my hometown. It was hot outside so I wore shorts and a halter top. I was talking with the old man across the street from where I grew up when suddenly his wife appeared. The first thing she said was that she couldn't imagine who that attractive teenage girl was that her husband was talking with. That teenage girl was me, and I'll be 54 years old next month.*"

CLAUDE HOWELL
— • • • —

age: 53
height: 5'5 1/2"

LOST 21 1/4 pounds of fat, **RESHAPED** her body by adding 8 pounds of muscle, and **TRIMMED** 5 inches off her waist, 5 3/8 inches off her hips, and 6 1/8 inches off her upper thighs in twelve weeks.

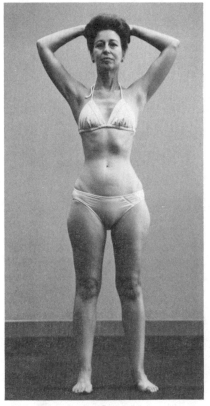 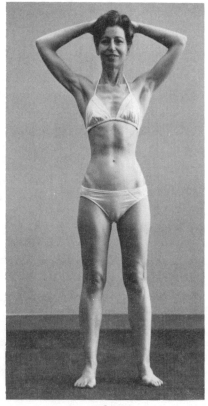

Before   **After**

••• UNDERSTAND MAINTENANCE CALORIES

On the Hot Hips and Fabulous Thighs maintenance plan, you must still be conscious of how many calories you eat each day. Only now, rather than trying to lose fat, you're trying to maintain it. Most women can maintain their existing level of fat on 1,500 to 2,200 calories a day. There is no simple method to determine in advance how many calories you will need to maintain your weight. Trial and error is the obvious course of action. Let's begin by examining the chart, Maintenance Guidelines for Calories.

Figuring out your maintenance level is accomplished by gradually adding calories from the four basic food groups to the 1,400 calorie-a-day diet you are already familiar with.

For example, try a certain level—say 1,600 calories a day—for two weeks. If your weight on the scale is still going down slightly,

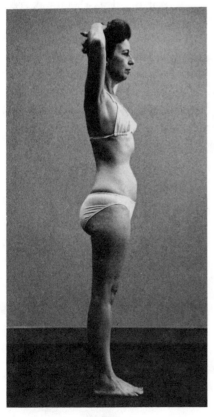
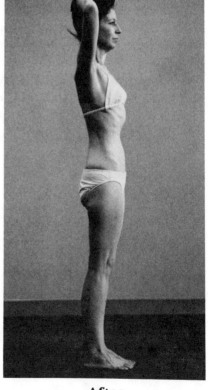

Before   **After**

raise your level to 1,800 a day for another two weeks. Your body weight then stabilizes. Now you know you have reached the upper limit of your maintenance caloric level.

It should not take you longer than a month to figure out your daily requirement for calories.

••• KEEP YOUR MUSCLES STRONG

You must continue to exercise your newly formed muscles or they will atrophy, or shrink, with disuse. Do not let this wasting away occur.

Strong and shapely muscles are important for Hot Hips and Fabulous Thighs. Firm, toned muscles are your best insurance policy against regaining your lost fat.

The primary difference between muscle-maintenance and muscle-building routines is that you do not need workouts as frequently in maintenance. In other words, muscle is hard to build, but easier to maintain.
To build muscle efficiently, you should exercise intensely three times per week. To maintain muscle, you only need to exercise half as often: three times in two weeks. You should still apply the super-slow guidelines that you've been applying for the last several months. You do not need to be as progressive in adding resistance or repetitions.

Keep in mind that more exercise is not necessarily better exercise. Better exercise is most often harder exercise. Apply this concept consistently and the shape of your hips and thighs may well exceed your goals.

···27···

Special Weekend Meals

$\vdots$

Many maintenance dieters, especially those who like to cook, ask for special weekend meals. They want low-calorie meals that are lavish, elegant, and stylish, the cuisine you might be presented at a plush health spa. Or the kind you would be pleased to serve weekend guests at your home.

I asked Brenda Hutchins once again to research the request and assemble some recipes that would even get Elizabeth Taylor excited. Brenda succeeded in royal fashion.

You can utilize any of the meals that follow as a part of your maintenance eating plan.

Bon appetit!

- **WEEKEND BREAKFAST ONE** (266 calories)
  Fruit Omelet Puff, Recipe #28 (179)
  1 slice reduced-calorie bread (40)
  1 teaspoon diet margarine (17)
  6 ounces decaffeinated swiss mocha, sugar-free (30)

- **WEEKEND BREAKFAST TWO** (260 calories)
  Strawberry Breakfast Crepes, Recipe #29 (134)
  2 slices wafer-thin bacon, cooked crisp and well drained (46)
  1 cup Hot Spiced Cran-Apple Cider, Recipe #30 (80)

- **WEEKEND LUNCH ONE** (348 calories)
  Weekend Party Pizza, Recipe #31 (213)
  Chocolate-Glazed Pear, Recipe #32 (135)
  Noncaloric beverage

- **WEEKEND LUNCH TWO** (350 calories)
  West Coast Minestrone, Recipe #33 (150)
  4 stone ground wheat crackers (56)
  1 slice reduced-calorie cheese (50)
  Pear Puff, Recipe #34 (94)
  Noncaloric beverage

- **WEEKEND DINNER ONE** (355 calories)
  Garlic Chicken, Recipe #35 (150)
  Dilled Green Bean & Potato Salad, Recipe #36 (95)
  1 slice reduced-calorie Italian bread (40)
  1 teaspoon diet margarine (17)
  Berries 'N' Cream, Recipe #37 (53)
  Noncaloric beverage

- **WEEKEND DINNER TWO** (355 calories)
  Grilled Swordfish in Pineapple Sauce, Recipe #38 (160)
  3 ounces steamed new potatoes, unpeeled (48)
  1 tablespoon non-fat plain yogurt (7)
  Chopped chives
  1/2 cup French-style green beans, steamed (16)
  Special Spinach Salad, Recipe #39 (44)
  Old-Fashioned Peach Cobbler, Recipe #40 (80)
  Noncaloric beverage

SPECIAL WEEKEND RECIPES

- *Recipe #28*

FRUIT OMELET PUFF
—————— • • • ——————

2   whole eggs, separated
2   egg whites
3   teaspoons granulated sugar
2   tablespoons unbleached all-purpose flour
$1/2$ teaspoon baking powder
1   teaspoon vanilla
$1/8$ teaspoon salt
$1/2$ cup skim milk
     Butter-flavor cooking spray
1   sweet red apple (3-inch diameter), quartered,
        cored, and cut into $1/2$-inch pieces
1   pear (3-inch × 2 $1/2$-inch diameter), quartered, cored,
        and cut into 2-inch pieces
2   teaspoons brown sugar
1   teaspoon fresh lemon juice
$1/4$ teaspoon ground cinnamon
2   tablespoons low-sugar raspberry preserves
2   teaspoons unsweetened apple juice

Preheat oven to 450 degrees. Beat all 4 egg whites with
3 teaspoons of sugar until they form soft peaks; set
aside.

Whisk together the egg yolks, flour, baking powder,
vanilla, salt, and three tablespoons of the milk until
well blended (5 to 7 minutes). Stir in half of the
egg-white mixture and then gently fold in the remaining
egg-mixture and milk, just until the mixture is blended;
do not overmix. Set the egg mixture aside.

Treat a large, ovenproof skillet with cooking spray
for 2 seconds and place over medium heat. Add the
apple, pear, brown sugar, lemon juice, and cinnamon;
cook the fruit until tender—about 5 minutes. Remove
skillet from the heat and pour egg mixture over the
fruit; smooth the top of the mixture with a spatula.

Place the skillet in a pre-heated oven and bake until the top is golden brown—about 10 to 15 minutes.

While the omelet is baking, mix the preserves and apple juice together in a small dish. When the omelet is ready, drizzle raspberry-apple syrup over the top; divide into quarters and serve immediately.

Yield: 4 servings
Calories: 179 per serving

• *Recipe #29*

STRAWBERRY BREAKFAST CREPES
• • •

8   crepes (recipe to follow)
8   ounces low-fat (1%) cottage cheese
2   tablespoons low-sugar orange marmalade (8
        calories/teaspoon)
     Ground cinnamon
     Strawberry Sauce (recipe to follow)

Yield: 8 crepes (2 crepes per serving)
Calories: 134 per serving

Note: If crepes were made in advance, preheat oven to 300 degrees. Spread crepes in a single layer on a baking sheet; cover with aluminum foil and bake for 3 to 5 minutes, until warm but not dried out.

Filling: Mix together the cottage cheese and low-sugar marmalade in a small mixing bowl and set aside.

Crepe Assembly: Fold 2 crepes in half and place on a serving plate with straight sides touching. Lift up tops of crepes and spread 2 tablespoons of cottage cheese mixture over each bottom half and sprinkle with cinnamon and fold down the tops of the crepes. Top each with 2 tablespoons Strawberry Sauce.

CREPE RECIPE

1	whole egg
2	egg whites
1 ¼	cups skim milk
¾	cup sifted, whole wheat flour
¼	cup sifted, unbleached white flour
2	teaspoons vegetable oil
1	teaspoon ground cinnamon
½	teaspoon vanilla
¼	teaspoon almond flavoring
1	teaspoon granulated sugar
	Butter-flavor cooking spray

Combine all ingredients except cooking spray in a food processor; blend ingredients for 1 minute. Pour into another container; cover and refrigerate overnight. (This allows flour particles to swell and soften so crepes are light in texture.)

Check the consistency of the batter before cooking; if thicker than heavy cream, add more skim milk, a teaspoonful at a time, until you have the proper consistency.

Coat the bottom of a 6-inch crepe pan with cooking spray; place over medium heat until just hot, not smoking. Put about 2 tablespoons of batter into pan; quickly tilt pan in all directions so batter covers pan in a thin film. Cook about one minute (underside should be golden).

Lift edge of crepe to check for doneness. Crepe is ready for flipping when it can be shaken loose. Flip and cook about 30 seconds on the other side. (This side is rarely more than spotty brown and is the side on which filling is placed.) Continue to cook crepes, and when necessary, remove pan from heat and re-coat with cooking spray.

When crepe is done, place on a towel to cool. Stack crepes between layers of waxed paper to prevent sticking. Stack crepes in batches of eight. Use immediately, or, allow to cool, wrap in air-tight container or storage bag, and refrigerate for up to 3 days or freeze for up to a month. (Frozen crepes should be defrosted in the refrigerator.) HINT: Crepes also make an elegant dessert, served filled with fruit or ice milk.

Yield: 32 crepes   **Calories:** 30 per crepe

STRAWBERRY SAUCE RECIPE

2   cups strawberries (fresh or frozen unsweetened, thawed)
¼   cup water
1½   tablespoons sugar
2   teaspoons cornstarch
¼   teaspoon almond extract

Combine strawberries, 3 tablespoons of water and 1½ tablespoons of sugar in a heavy saucepan; cook over medium heat until strawberries are soft. Dissolve cornstarch in remaining tablespoon of water; add to strawberries and continue cooking, stirring constantly, until sauce thickens. Stir in almond extract; remove from heat. Serve warm or chilled. HINT: This sauce is delicious over ice milk or stirred into plain yogurt or applesauce.

Yield: 2 cups   **Calories:** 6 per tablespoon

• *Recipe #30*

HOT SPICED CRAN-APPLE CIDER
——————————— •●• ———————————

2   cups apple cider
2   cups low-calorie cranberry juice cocktail
1   cinnamon stick
4   whole cloves
4   whole coriander seeds

Combine all ingredients in a saucepan and bring to a boil. Reduce heat and simmer uncovered for 4 to 5 minutes. Serve in a pre-heated mug.

Yield: 4 8-ounce servings **Calories:** 80 per serving

• *Recipe #31*

WEEKEND PARTY PIZZA
• • •

Olive oil-flavor cooking spray
1/2 cup chopped onion
1 1/2 cups Basil-Spiced Tomato Sauce (recipe to follow)
1 teaspoon fresh oregano or 1/2 teaspoon dried
4 8-inch flour tortillas
1 cup grated part-skim mozzarella cheese
2/3 cup fresh mushrooms, sliced
12 jumbo black olives, pitted and diced

Preheat oven to 350 degrees. Coat the bottom of a nonstick skillet with cooking spray; place over medium heat until just hot, not smoking. Add onion and sauté for 3 to 5 minutes, until translucent. Add tomato sauce and oregano and cook for 1 minute; remove from heat.

Arrange tortillas in a single layer on a baking sheet; bake for 4 to 5 minutes (until crisp). Remove from oven and spread each tortilla with one-fourth tomato sauce mixture; top each with one-fourth mozzarella, mushrooms and olives. Continue baking for 5 minutes or until cheese melts. Serve immediately.

Yield: 4 servings
Calories: 213 each

BASIL-SPICED TOMATO SAUCE RECIPE

Olive oil-flavor cooking spray
1 garlic clove, minced
2 tablespoons chopped chives
1 cup canned tomatoes, drained and diced
1 tablespoon chopped fresh basil

Coat a nonstick skillet with cooking spray; place over medium heat until just hot, not smoking. Sauté garlic and chives until tender; add tomatoes. Lower heat and simmer for 5 minutes. Stir in basil and heat through; remove from heat.

Yield: 4 servings   **Calories:** 19 per serving

• *Recipe #32*

CHOCOLATE-GLAZED PEAR
• • •

4   medium pears (about 6 1/2 ounces each)
1   tablespoon lemon juice
4   cups water
    Chocolate Glaze (recipe to follow)
    Fresh mint sprigs (optional)

Peel pears; core from bottom, cutting to but *not* through stem end. Brush pears with lemon juice to prevent browning. (Reserve any leftover juice.)

Combine remaining lemon juice with water in a large saucepan; bring water to a boil. Place pears in saucepan (in upright position); cover; reduce heat and simmer 12 to 15 minutes or until tender.

Remove pears with slotted spoon and allow to drain. Spoon 1 1/2 tablespoons Chocolate Sauce in a dessert dish; top each with a poached pear. Drizzle 1/2 tablespoon Chocolate Sauce over each pear. Garnish each with fresh mint springs, if desired.

Yield: 4 servings
Calories: 135 per serving

CHOCOLATE SAUCE RECIPE

1/2   cup water
1   tablespoon sugar
1   teaspoon cornstarch
1   teaspoon vanilla extract
3 1/2 tablespoons sugar-free chocolate flavor mix
2   tablespoons dry white wine

Combine first 4 ingredients in a medium saucepan, ˙ stirring until smooth. Cook over medium heat, stirring constantly, until smooth and thickened. Remove from heat; whisk in chocolate flavor mix, one tablespoon at a time. Stir in wine; allow to cool. HINT: Chocolate Sauce is heavenly over ice milk or Breakfast Crepes (as a dessert) stuffed with ice milk or fruit.

Yield: ½ cup
Calories: 17 per tablespoon

● *Recipe #33*

WEST COAST MINESTRONE
● ● ●

    Olive oil-flavor cooking spray
1   teaspoon olive oil
½ cup chopped onion
½ cup chopped carrot
½ cup chopped celery
1   garlic clove, minced
1   (14½-ounce) can tomatoes, drained and chopped
1   (7½-ounce) can chicken broth
3   cups water
10 spinach leaves, washed, drained and coarsely
      chopped
1   (15½-ounce) can kidney beans, drained
3   ounces (dry weight) vermicelli (broken in half)
2   tablespoons chopped fresh parsley
¼ cup grated Parmesan cheese
    Salt and pepper

Coat the bottom of a 4-quart pot with cooking spray and add olive oil. Sauté chopped vegetables and minced garlic over medium heat for 3 to 5 minutes, stirring often. Add chicken broth and water; bring to a boil. Lower heat and simmer, uncovered, for 25 minutes. Add spinach and kidney beans and bring soup to a boil. Add the vermicelli, lower heat and cook until *al dente* (about 5 to 7 minutes). Serve in large heated soup bowls, sprinkle each serving with 1 tablespoon Parmesan cheese, and add salt and pepper to taste.

Yield: 4 servings   **Calories:** 150 per serving

● **Recipe #34**

PEAR PUFF
————————● ● ●————————

2 sheets commercial frozen phyllo pastry, thawed
3 medium (about 6 ½ ounces) pears, peeled and
   chopped, or 6 canned juice-packed pear halves,
   well-drained
2 tablespoons brown sugar
   Butter-flavor cooking spray
1 teaspoon ground cinnamon
4 teaspoons diet margarine
1 tablespoon powdered sugar

Divide each sheet of phyllo dough in half. (Keep each
phyllo sheet covered until needed.)

Combine chopped pears and brown sugar; toss to
coat evenly. Place one half-sheet of phyllo on a damp
towel (keep remaining phyllo covered). Lightly coat
phyllo sheet with cooking spray and fold in half
lengthwise and spray again. Place one-fourth pear
mixture at base of sheet, sprinkle with cinnamon, and
top with 1 teaspoon diet margarine. Fold the right
bottom corner over filling, making a triangle. Continue
folding back and forth into a triangle to end of sheet.
Repeat process with each remaining phyllo sheet and
pear mixture. Keep triangles covered before baking.

Place triangles, seam-side down, on a nonstick
baking sheet treated with cooking spray. Bake at 400
degrees for 15 minutes or until golden brown. Remove
from oven and dust with powdered sugar.

Yield: 4 servings
Calories: 94 per puff

• *Recipe #35*

GARLIC CHICKEN
———————————•●•———————————

4   boneless, skinless chicken breasts (about 5 ounces
      raw weight each)
1   garlic clove, minced
      Juice of 1 lemon
1   teaspoon olive oil
2   tablespoons diet Italian dressing
$1/2$ tablespoon fresh thyme or $1/4$ teaspoon dried
      Salt and pepper to taste
      Olive oil-flavor cooking spray

Combine all ingredients except spray in a bowl; toss to coat evenly. Cover and refrigerate for at least 2 hours.

Preheat broiler. Coat broiler pan with cooking spray; remove chicken from marinade and place on broiler pan. Broil 4 to 5 minutes on each side, or until cooked but not dry.

Yield: 4 servings   **Calories:** 150 per serving

• *Recipe #36*

DILLED GREEN BEAN & POTATO SALAD
———————————•●•———————————

1 $1/2$ cups French-style green beans
10   ounces small new potatoes, scrubbed
1   hard-cooked egg, chopped
1   small green onion, sliced (including tops)
$1/2$ cup celery, sliced
$2/3$ cup non-fat plain yogurt
1   teaspoon Dijon mustard
1   teaspoon chopped fresh dill
      Salt and pepper to taste
      Paprika

Steam green beans and new potatoes until tender. Let potatoes cool and cut into $1/4$-inch pieces (do not peel).

Combine beans, potatoes, and remaining ingredients. Toss to mix, sprinkle with paprika, and chill.

Yield: 4 servings   **Calories:** 95 per serving

- **Recipe #37**

BERRIES 'N' CREAM
· · ·

1/2 cup low-fat vanilla yogurt
1/4 teaspoon almond flavoring
1/8 teaspoon ground nutmeg
2 cups strawberries (fresh or frozen unsweetened, thawed)
2 tablespoons blueberries (fresh or frozen unsweetened, thawed)

Mix yogurt, flavoring, and nutmeg together in a small bowl.

Place 1/2 cup strawberries in each of 4 dessert dishes, top with 2 tablespoons yogurt mixture, and garnish with 1/2 tablespoon blueberries. Chill.

Yield: 4 servings   **Calories:** 53 per serving

- **Recipe #38**

GRILLED SWORDFISH
IN PINEAPPLE SAUCE
· · ·

Butter-flavor cooking spray
2 tablespoons finely chopped green onion
2 tablespoons chopped fresh tarragon or 2 teaspoons dried
1/2 cup canned chicken broth
1/4 cup pineapple juice
1 1/2 teaspoons cornstarch, mixed with
1 tablespoon cold water
1/4 teaspoon garlic salt
Freshly ground black pepper
1 pound swordfish steak, trimmed and cut into quarters
4 slices pineapple (fresh or juice-packed, canned)

Coat a broiler pan with cooking spray and preheat broiler.

Coat a saucepan with cooking spray; place over

medium heat just until hot, not smoking. Add the green onion and cook until tender (1 to 2 minutes). Add tarragon, chicken broth, pineapple juice, cornstarch mixture, garlic salt, and pepper; whisk continuously and bring mixture to a boil. Reduce heat to low and simmer sauce until it thickens (about 2 to 3 minutes). Remove from heat and set aside.

Rinse fish under cold running water and pat them dry with paper towels; season steaks with garlic salt and pepper, then spray them lightly with cooking spray. Broil the steaks until flesh is opaque and feels firm to touch—3 to 4 minutes each side.

When fish is nearly done, reheat sauce over low heat. Serve fish immediately, topped with warm sauce and garnished with pineapple slices.

Yield: 4 servings   **Calories:** 160 per serving

* *Recipe #39*

SPECIAL SPINACH SALAD
— • • • —

½   pound young tender spinach leaves, washed and
      patted dry, stems removed
1   large carrot (use potato peeler and form carrot
      curls, pinned with toothpicks and placed in ice
      water)
⅓   package enoki mushrooms, root-ends trimmed
1   cup cherry tomatoes, washed and halved
½   cup green onion, diced (including top)
4   tablespoons diet Italian dressing
4   teaspoons grated Parmesan cheese

Divide spinach leaves among four salad plates. Remove toothpicks from carrot curls and place about 5 or 6 mushroom stems in each curl; arrange curls over the spinach leaves. Place ¼ cherry tomato halves and green onions on each plate. Top each salad with 1 tablespoon diet Italian dressing and 1 teaspoon cheese. Serve at once.

Yield: 4 servings   **Calories:** 44 per serving

● *Recipe #40*

OLD-FASHIONED PEACH COBBLER
● ● ●

2   large peaches (3-inch, 6-ounce) or 2 cups canned,
        juice-packed
1/8 teaspoon ground cinnamon
1   tablespoon brown sugar
1   tablespoon diet margarine, melted
        Butter-flavor cooking spray
1/2 cup Home Granola, from Recipe #1

Preheat oven to 350 degrees.

Peel and quarter peaches, then cut into 1/4-inch
wedges. Add next 3 ingredients; toss to mix.

Coat 4 small baking dishes with cooking spray;
divide peach mixture among the dishes and bake for 7
to 9 minutes. Sprinkle 2 tablespoons granola over each
cobbler and return to oven for 3 more minutes. Serve
piping hot.

Yield: 4 servings
Calories: 80 per serving

···28···

Backsliding Forward

$\vdots$

You may have stuck to the diet strictly for weeks. Then you wrecked it one day as you walked by a donut shop. Fifteen minutes later you'd wolfed down almost a dozen!

You may be progressing nicely with your strength-training routine. An unexpected emergency, however, causes you to miss several workouts.

Now you feel guilty. You broke the diet. You sloughed off on your exercise. You might as well forget the whole program and go back to your old ways.

Stop! Don't let yourself fall into this senseless, destructive trap. Guilt saps your motivation and confidence.

Furthermore, such thinking indicates only a short-term goal. True power revolves around the realization that permanent fat loss is a long-term project that is bound to have a few ups and downs.

Expect to backslide occasionally. You're only human, right? There is no disgrace in backsliding. The disgrace lies in letting a lapse get you so discouraged that you quit trying. You must move forward.

●● PREPARE FOR LAPSES

Lapses usually follow urges. When you saw or smelled the donuts, you had an urge or craving for one, then another, and another. If you recognize urges for what they are—certainly not indications of true hunger—you can turn them into signals for corrective action.

169

Urges can be compared to ocean waves. Both formulate slowly, pick up momentum, come to a crest, break, and subside gently on the shore.

You might believe urges come on like monsters that can be satisfied only by giving in, by submission, by eating. Caving in to an urge results in more guilt, which results in more urges, more often, with more inertia behind them. If you ride the wave, if you let it crest and pass, it will weaken and splash onto shore. Moreover, the next one will be easier to ride.

There will always be urges—the urge for a donut, a second helping, a bowl of ice cream, an alcoholic drink. The waves roll in most furiously during high tide, meaning your high-risk situations.

Being in control requires identifying the oncoming wave in time to prepare for it. You then have to be able to ride it out. Detecting its approach—and knowing how to get on top—makes you a skilled urge surfer. Either without the other results in a lot of wipeouts.

Anticipate your high-tide times by making a list of your high-risk situations. These will be readily apparent if you keep a brief written record of when and where you eat for several days. These patterns will clearly emerge.

••• SUBSTITUTE ALTERNATIVE ACTIVITIES

Are you at high risk when in the house alone just before the kids come home from school? Is it at night in front of the TV, subject to a billion-dollar advertising industry urging you to consume food? Are you a stress eater, using calories to douse the flames of frustration? Do you cope with boredom by pampering yourself with food your body doesn't need?

Ride the wave of eating urges by having another list of alternative activities. This list might include such things as taking a walk, shopping, exercising, doing your fingernails, brushing your teeth, reading a fitness publication, taking a bath, taking a drive, refinishing furniture, or working in the garden.

Simply substitute the activity for the urge. Instead of eating a donut, do your fingernails. Instead of eating a bowl of ice cream, take a bath.

*"**I**'ve been on a maintenance plan for over a year. The concept of backsliding forward has made a big difference with my ups and downs. The key to keeping fat off, in my opinion, is learning how to deal with cravings. Staying busy with fitness activities has helped me bury these cravings for certain foods."*

DIANE TRAVIS
————————— • • • —————————

age: 44
height: 5'4"

LOST 24 ½ pounds of fat, **RESHAPED** her body by adding 7 pounds of muscle, and **TRIMMED** 4 ⅝ inches off her waist, 2 ⅞ inches off her hips, and 5 ⅜ inches off her upper thighs in twelve weeks.

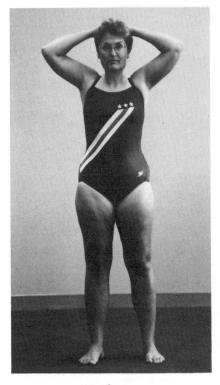 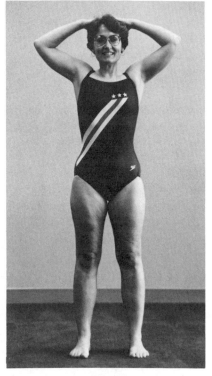

Before   **After**

••• USE IT OR LOSE IT

If you've lapsed in regard to exercise, the remedy will depend on the length of the lapse. It takes about the same amount of time to lose strength as it takes you to gain it. If you increase the strength of your hip and thigh muscles by 50 percent in six weeks, then it will take you six weeks to lose that strength—given that you do no exercise during that time period.

Thus, for each workout you skip, you must back up a workout in restarting your exercise.

Miss four workouts, then back up four workouts. But take note. Your muscles retain a memory of strength. It's always easier to exercise back to your previous condition than it was originally. Unless it's been many months, you're still ahead of where you started.

Don't lose it. Use it!

···29···

Tanning: Shedding Light on the Issue

We've all heard about the problems related to exposure to the sun. The sun causes your skin to age prematurely, and too much can lead to skin cancer.

On the other hand, a suntan makes a woman's body—especially her legs—look more attractive. Competitive bodybuilders, those men and women who flex and pose their muscles under stage lights, know that a tan accentuates their definition and curves. It can do the same for you.

One experienced bodybuilding judge explained it like this: "You get a dent in the fender of a white car, nobody notices. Get one in a dark car, people see it from blocks down the street." Dents in fenders are similar to the curves provided by shapely muscles.

There are no 100 percent safe ways to get a suntan. But there are guidelines to follow to make your tanning as safe as possible.

··• DO NOT BURN

Dermatologists are in agreement that you should absolutely avoid getting a sunburn. Melanoma, the most dangerous of the skin diseases, is seldom found on the face. It is usually found on the backs of men and legs of women, indicating that infrequent and sudden exposure may be the determining factor. The short, ultraviolet beta rays (UVB) present when the sun is high and most intense do the most damage. If possible, avoid sunning between the hours of 11:00 a.m. and 2:00 p.m.

It is recommended that initially you use a sunscreen with a sun-protection factor (SPF) of 15. The SPF is a measure of the level of protection from UVB you are getting. A sunscreen with SPF 15 allows you to stay in the sun without burning 15 times longer than you'd be able to if you weren't wearing any sunscreen. It provides 95 percent protection against UVB.

Most dermatologists say that SPFs of more than 15 are overkill. Not only are these megasunscreens costly, but they're more likely to cause skin irritation because they contain more chemicals.

Even with sunscreens you should keep your exposure gradual. Do not rush it. It usually takes from ten days to two weeks of progressive daily exposure to get a pleasing tan on your legs.

•• TANNING BOOTHS

Millions of people in the United States regularly use tanning booths. Yet we know very little about the long-range effects of artificial tanning. Manufacturers of tanning beds claim that because the lamps used in these products produce the longer ultraviolet rays (UVA), they are safer than natural sunlight. The UVA rays penetrate more deeply into the skin without causing as much surface burning.

That deeper penetration may make the UVA rays potentially more dangerous. No one knows for sure. Some dermatologists, however, say that UVA rays affect the body's immune system and lower resistance to disease.

If you use a tanning booth, be sure to wear the goggles provided. Exposing your eyes to high doses of ultraviolet light can lead to cataracts, and closing your eyes offers no protection against it. Always use goggles.

•• SUNLESS TANNING PRODUCTS

There are three kinds of sunless, or artificial, tanning products available: a temporary bronzer, a paint-on skin dye, and a longer-lasting stain that reacts with your skin.

Bronzers work like ordinary makeup powders. They contain washable pigments that make the skin look tan when they're applied.

Paint-on skin dyes are a blend of various coloring agents that are sponged onto the body. They wear off gradually over several weeks. Two of the most popular brands used by bodybuilders are Dy-O-Derm and Pro Tan.

Skin stains contain an ingredient called dihydroxyacetone, which causes a chemical reaction on the skin. The resulting color can range from orange to yellow and can last for two weeks. Even with improvements, many users continue to assert that the color is not natural looking.

••• GUIDELINES FOR TANNING OR COLORING YOUR SKIN

Using the sun:
- Use sunscreens in the beginning.
- Don't rush it. Expose your skin slowly to avoid burning.
- Avoid the most intense midday sun.
- Check with your doctor if you're taking prescription drugs. Some drugs increase your sensitivity to the sun.

Using a tanning bed:
- Deal with respected, experienced salons.
- Start with short exposures.
- Wear goggles. Closing your eyes offers no protection.
- Do not go beyond recommended time limits.

Using a dye:
- Cleanse the skin thoroughly and apply a moisturizer before applying the dye.
- Apply evenly with a makeup sponge. The dye will stain your hands and fingernails.
- Spread very light coats over your knees, ankles, wrists, and elbows.
- Allow dye to air dry.
- Reapply as desired. Each application will promote further darkening.
- Continue to use moisturizer for skin dryness.

••• KEEP IT LIGHT

A light tan can be almost as eye-catching as a dark tan—and it's certainly healthier. Besides, the ease or difficulty with which you tan, as well as how dark you can get, is genetically determined.

If you decide to tan your body, play it safe.

And keep it light!

···*30*···

Diet-Related Problems

$\vdots$

Many of the questions I get from women concern problems that appear during or after dieting. Here's a guide to help you understand and combat some of them.

••• BRUISING

Black and blue marks often appear on the hips and thighs of dieting and exercising women without trauma significant enough to merit the size of the bruise. Such bruising is the result of an increased level of estrogen circulating in the body, which somehow weakens the walls of the capillaries and causes them to break under the slightest pressure. When this happens, blood escapes and a bruise occurs.

Estrogen is broken down in the liver, and so is fat. When you are dieting, your liver preferentially breaks down the fat, leaving a lot more estrogen in the bloodstream. It may be helpful to supplement your diet with 100 milligrams of vitamin C per day to help toughen the walls of the capillaries.

••• COLD SENSITIVITY

Some dieters complain about being cold much of the time. Even during the summer, air conditioning can bring on the chills. So can drinking the recommended amounts of ice water each day.

Much of your fat is located right under your skin and acts as insulation. Once you begin to lose this insulation, it's no wonder that you become more sensitive to cold. Your fingers, toes, even the tip of your nose can be affected.

The cure is to dress warmly, especially during the winter. Also, it helps to realize that a little bit of shivering is one of the best ways for your body to burn calories.

••• CONSTIPATION

The cause of constipation is usually decreased food intake and increased water loss. The cure is to drink lots of water and consume the recommended fruits, vegetables, breads, and cereals.

••• DIARRHEA

Women who suffer diarrhea on the Hot Hips and Fabulous Thighs diet are usually allergic to milk. They suffer from lactose intolerance. Lactose intolerance occurs when you don't have enough of a certain enzyme in your stomach to digest the lactose in milk. When you consume milk or milk products, you develop gas, abdominal distension, cramps, and sometimes diarrhea.

Lactose intolerance does not have to signal an end to your milk-drinking days. You can buy the missing enzyme (lactose), in tablet or capsule form, to take orally when eating dairy products, or put enzyme drops directly into milk before drinking it. Or, you can purchase lactose-free dairy products from your specialty grocer.

••• DRY MOUTH

More water is the cure for dry mouth. Fat acts as a portable water tank, since your fat is composed of 20 percent water. As you become leaner you lose this potential source of water. Thus, you have to drink more and more water on a daily basis as you become leaner and leaner.

Drinking more water is also a cure for dry skin.

••• HALITOSIS (BAD BREATH)

Halitosis is often caused by the metabolic state in which your body burns fat for energy. This should not be alarming. The slight unpleasant odor can be combated by eating smaller meals more often and, once again, by drinking more water.

*"**P**revious diets that I've been on always left me dehydrated, constipated, tired, and listless. I've suffered none of these during the Hot Hips and Fabulous Thighs program. I feel better than ever."*

KATHY BENNETT
—————————•••—————————
age: 36
height: 5′5³/₄″

LOST 18¹/₄ pounds of fat, **RESHAPED** her body by adding 4¹/₂ pounds of muscle, and **TRIMMED** 3⁵/₈ inches off her waist, 2³/₄ inches off her hips, and 5 inches off her upper thighs in six weeks.

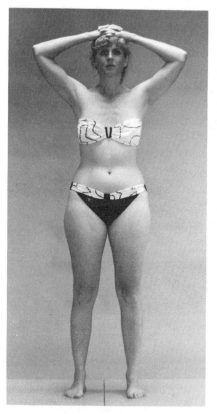 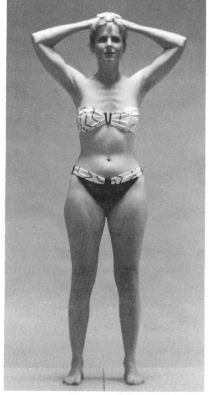

Before   **After**

If, on the other hand, your breath has a heavy fruity or acidic odor, your body may be burning both fat and muscle as a source of energy. This is an unhealthy state. Your diet is probably too low in calories or carbohydrates. Check your food weighing and measuring, as well as calorie counting, and make appropriate adjustments.

••• INSOMNIA

Insomnia is the inability to fall asleep, or once asleep, to stay asleep. It may be caused by too much caffeine. Check your beverages, such as coffee, tea, and diet sodas. Try the caffeine-free versions, and drink more plain water.

Some women on the Hot Hips and Fabulous Thighs program actually find that after losing a significant amount of fat they require less sleep per night. Try to reduce your sleeping habits and see if it helps.

••• MUSCLE CRAMPS

Cramps are painful muscle spasms which occur most often in feet, calves, or fingers. They are usually caused by dehydration— which means you are *not* drinking enough water. For immediate relief, slowly extend or stretch the involved muscles in the opposite direction of the cramp. Hold this position gently for 20 to 30 seconds.

···31···

Frequently Asked Questions

:

Two chapters of questions and answers should add the finishing touches to this program.

•• WHY NO AEROBICS?

Q. *Why are no aerobics included on the Hot Hips and Fabulous Thighs program?*

A. To answer this question, we must examine three definitions of aerobic.

First, aerobic generally relates to an activity that entails an increased involvement of the heart and lungs for a prolonged time. If the heart rate doubles when you run across a busy intersection, and then returns to normal after a few seconds or minutes, the activity is anaerobic or not aerobic. If the activity is continued long enough at a pace to sustain an elevated heart rate for many minutes, then it is said to be aerobic.

Second, biochemists classify our energy-producing metabolic pathways as aerobic and anaerobic. Aerobic refers to the presence of oxygen, whereas anaerobic means without oxygen.

Third, to many people aerobics mean whole-body dance movements that are performed in a group setting to popular music. Jacki Sorensen, Jane Fonda, and Kathy Smith promote this type of aerobics.

The Nautilus routines recommended on the Hot Hips and Fabulous Thighs program can involve your heart, lungs, and metabolic system aerobically—according to the first and second definitions. To do this, however, you must be skilled in the use of Nautilus equipment, be strong enough to elevate your heart rate from 70 to 85 percent of your maximum level, and be enduring enough to move quickly from one machine to the next in fifteen seconds or less.

During the last two weeks of the program, it is easily possible to keep your heart rate at 70 to 85 percent of your maximum level for 15 to 20 minutes, which satisfies the major requirement for cardiovascular endurance. During the super-slow workout, your leg and arm muscles (depending on the specific exercise) are involved anaerobically. But your core torso muscles—the abdominal and erector spinae, for example—are working aerobically because they are required for stabilization during each exercise.

I do not recommend that you combine Nautilus training with aerobic dancing movements, described in the third definition. Aerobic dancing—and other activities such as running, swimming, cycling, and racquetball—do not contribute significantly to the fat-loss process. In fact, when added to the Nautilus program they can actually retard the loss of fat.

Fat loss is retarded in two ways. Too much repetitive activity prevents maximum muscle building by using up your recovery ability. A well-rested recovery ability is necessary for muscle growth. Too much activity—especially if you're on a' reduced-calorie diet—causes you to get the blahs and quickly lose your enthusiasm. If this happens, you're sure to break your diet.

The primary purpose of the program is to lose fat in the most effective and most efficient manner. Fat loss is prioritized and maximized by building muscle at the same time. The muscle-building process is optimized by a well-rested recovery ability, which necessitates keeping your strenuous and moderately strenuous activities to a bare minimum.

Once you get your body fat to a low level, you can add other activities—and I encourage you to do so—to your weekly fitness schedule. Then, if you wish to do both, perform Nautilus and aerobics on the same day and rest the day after. For now, follow the program exactly as directed.

Q. *So you're saying that the Nautilus program already in-volves aerobic conditioning?*

A. Yes, the recommended super-slow exercise certainly has the capacity to provide aerobic conditioning—if you are skilled enough, strong enough, and enduring enough to perform each exercise properly. Doing each exercise slowly and then moving quickly between machines will keep your heart rate elevated to the desired level for 15 to 20 minutes. It also works your core torso muscles continuously for the duration of the workout. Further-more, because the exercise is performed slowly and smoothly, it is very safe compared to aerobic dancing and jogging.

•• FREEHAND ROUTINES

Q. *Do the freehand routines in this book supply adequate aer-obic conditioning?*

A. No, not as adequately as do the Nautilus routines. The recom-mended freehand routines are not designed to supply aerobic con-ditioning. They are designed to provide effective muscular stimulation to the hips and thighs.

Once again, after you've lost your excessive fat you can include aerobic conditioning in your program.

•• FUN OR TORTURE?

Q. *Many advertisements for fitness centers lead me to believe that exercising is fun. Yet you say high-intensity super-slow ex-ercise is the opposite of fun. What's the truth?*

A. High-intensity super-slow exercise challenges the human body. It acts as a stimulus which forces the body to overcompen-sate and get stronger. Soon, however, the body adapts and the stimulus must be made more intense.

Such exercise would only be fun to people who enjoy high levels of physiological stress. The vast majority of people do not enjoy the uncomfortable feelings that occur when muscles are repetitively stretched and contracted and the heart and lungs strain to provide large amounts of oxygen to the working muscles. When exercise becomes fun, it usually produces only mainte-nance results.

"It's torture, but it works," is the theme of a very successful fitness center in California. While super-slow exercise may not be torture, it is certainly rather limited in the fun area.

The fun part of super-slow exercise comes when you have reached a level of fitness that you are satisfied with. Then you can stay at that level with only maintenance training.

The fun part comes when you see the changes in the mirror and the people you care about start noticing and complimenting you on your physical appearance.

•• PHYSICAL ATTRACTIVENESS

Q. *I'm upset that it is the outside appearance of a woman's body that primarily attracts a man. Can't something be done to correct this situation?*

A. Rest assured that there are other people who are concerned as well. Being upset, however, does not change the long-standing social behavior of most Americans.

A recent issue of *Glamour* magazine reported the results of a survey which asked women the following question: "Have you ever felt people responded to you solely on the basis of your looks?"

"Yes," said a resounding 92 percent of the women who answered the survey.

"I've been rejected and even ostracized because of my physical appearance," wrote one concerned woman. "It seems that being overweight cancels five years of college and fluency in four languages."

"I'm fairly attractive," wrote another woman, "and at times become disgusted with men who tell me, 'You're very attractive, and I'd like to get to know you better.' What ever happened to intelligence and charm?"

Intelligence and charm are still desirable attributes, but according to the research of Dr. Ellen Berscheid, professor of psychology at the University of Minnesota, it does appear that they have taken a back seat to physical beauty. Do not underestimate the importance of how you look. The decade of the 1990s seems greatly influenced by a new wave of people who are interested in beautiful bodies.

*"**B**efore this program, I never did any type of muscle-building exercise. I didn't believe I needed it. Was I wrong.*

"I've seen the effects that super-slow exercise has on my muscles. Now, I'm a believer!"

KATHRYN COOK
•••
age: 31
height: 5'3¼"

LOST 15½ pounds of fat, **RESHAPED** her body by adding 5 pounds of muscle, and **TRIMMED** 4⅜ inches off her waist, 1¾ inches off her hips, and 2¾ inches off her upper thighs in six weeks.

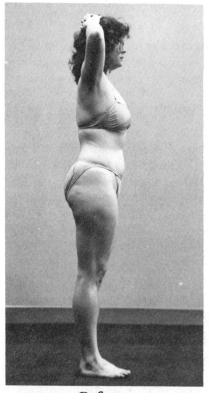
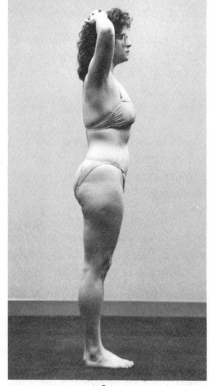

Before   **After**

Most people have little control over the social behavior of others. But you can try to understand the reasoning behind some of the behavior, whether you agree with it or not, and intelligently work with it to reach your goals.

••• STRETCHING AND FLEXIBILITY

Q. *I've always liked doing stretching movements to improve my flexibility. Can I supplement the Hot Hips and Fabulous Thighs program with stretching?*

A. For years, stretching movements have been used almost as a cure-all. Women have been told that stretching will improve their flexibility, firm and shape their body, reduce fat, and prevent injuries. As a result, women by the thousands stretch their bodies in organized classes at local clubs or in front of television instructors at home.

Most women are attracted to stretching movements simply because they are easy, fun, and social, especially since large groups can be directed in the same movements in unison. This is certainly acceptable. But the facts show that the potential physiological benefits from stretching programs are limited and vastly overrated.

Flexibility is defined as the range of movement of a body segment around a joint or group of joints. Stretching performed slowly and smoothly does improve a person's flexibility. Women, because of their hormones and body composition, are generally more flexible than men. This is especially true of a woman's lower body. Yet most women seem to concentrate on movements that stretch the muscles of their hips and thighs. They mistakenly believe that stretching strengthens and firms their muscles, which it does not; that stretching lengthens their muscles, which it does not; or that stretching reduces the fatty deposits on their hips and thighs, which it does not.

Furthermore, there are not conclusive *data* that increased flexibility prevents injuries. Research does show that muscular strength throughout fullrange joint movements is the primary factor that prevents injury.

You need to emphasize super-slow strength training much more than stretching movements. It is the strength of your muscles, not the flexibility of your joints, that contributes to a shapely figure.

••• AFRAID OF LARGE MUSCLES

Q. *Although the women you feature in this book don't have large muscles, I still fear I might get them from the type of exercise you recommend. Can you assure me that I won't get large muscles from the Hot Hips and Fabulous Thighs program?*

A. Yes. You will not get large muscles from this program. Building large muscles requires two conditions. First, the individual must have long muscles and short tendons. Second, an abundance of male hormones, particularly testosterone, must be present in the bloodstream. Women almost never have either of these conditions.

Under no circumstances could 99.99 percent of American women develop excessively large muscles. High-intensity, super-slow exercise will make your muscles larger—but not excessively large—and larger muscles along with less fat will turn your body into firmer and more shapely flesh.

Q. *What about all those women athletes with large muscles?*

A. It should be understood that most women do not have the genetic potential to develop unusually large muscles. Women, as well as men, with large muscles are genetic rarities. The vast majority of women involved in Olympic and professional sports have slim, well-toned bodies. It is unfortunate that certain photographs and publicity have led people to believe that women athletes with large muscles are the rule rather than the rare exception.

During the recent Olympic games, there were many very tall women playing basketball. One Russian player was 7 feet 2 inches tall. A teammate of hers measured 6 feet 8 inches tall. Most of the women on the medal-winning teams were over 6 feet.

After watching several Olympic basketball games, a woman might assume that bouncing a ball would make her taller. She might try various ball-bouncing routines with no success and conclude that bouncing a ball had no effect on increasing her height. She might also realize that if she grew in height it would be because of her genetic inheritance and not her activities.

The same is true for the very few women with large muscles. They have inherited above-average length muscles and above-average levels of male hormones. They have the ability to develop larger and more defined muscles than the typical woman. These few women will be larger and stronger than the average woman even if they never exercise or take part in sports.

If a woman who had all the genetic capabilities actually did develop unsightly muscles, she could go without exercise for several weeks and her muscles would shrink. Muscles are made to be used. If they are not used, they atrophy.

More Questions and Answers: Varicose Veins, Sweating, and Whirlpool Baths

·· • TANNING ACCELERATORS

Q. *In the chapter on tanning, you failed to mention the use of tanning accelerators. Are they helpful?*

A. The active ingredient in these products is tyrosine, an amino acid that may hasten tanning in some people. If you don't mind paying their high price, they may prove somewhat helpful. For the most part, however, the tan accelerators are simply moisturizers.

·· • VARICOSE VEINS

Q. *What are varicose veins and will this program benefit them?*

A. Varicose veins are bulging, twisted, and knotted veins that are usually located right under the skin. While they frequently occur in pregnant women, they appear in other women and men as well. Most often they develop in the legs, although they can surface in other places like the anal area (hemorrhoids) and the genital area. Their presence is due to two factors. One, many pregnancies contribute to a generally weakened condition of the veins in the legs if the pressure created by the baby cuts off circulation. Two, a tendency toward varicose veins can be genetic. In such a case, the individual probably inherited a tendency toward inelasticity in the vein walls.

In both instances, however, the results are the same: There is a weakness or malfunction within the flaplike valves of the vein. As the weight of the blood on the vein wall increases, the vein bulges, and after long stretching, it loses its elasticity and finally becomes elongated, twisted, and knotted.

The Hot Hips and Fabulous Thighs program can help varicose veins. Repeated contractions of the leg muscles milk the blood out of the lower body and propel it upward toward the heart. Everyone can benefit by maintaining strength in the hip and thigh muscles. The strong, firm muscles around the deep veins help provide external support and protection from overstretching and damage.

Q. *Can varicose veins be prevented?*

A. If you have a genetic predisposition for varicose veins, you probably will not be able to prevent them. These measures, however, will help minimize them:

- Avoid standing for long periods. If you must stand, wear lightweight support stockings. When standing at your job, at a party, or in line, flex your toes every few minutes and then rise slowly on your tiptoes.
- Do not sit for long periods, especially with your legs crossed. When sitting, elevate your legs or change their position. On long train, plane, or bus trips, walk about every half hour. On long car trips, switch drivers frequently, or stop for light exercise every hour, if possible.
- Discard tight garments that constrict your legs: girdles, garters, and knee-high stockings. High boots with elastic around the tops are especially bad.
- Keep your body fat within a normal range.
- Maintain strong muscles.

••• SPIDER VEINS

Q. *Are these small spider veins on my legs the same as varicose veins?*

A. No. These small spider-weblike clusters on your legs are usually caused by enlargement of a group of tiny capillaries in the skin. They are disturbing to look at but they are *not* varicose veins, merely a variation of normal veins. They are thought to be influenced by female hormones and occasionally appear more prominent following use of birth control pills.

Q. *Is there any treatment for spider veins?*

A. These veins are best left alone, or, if especially prominent, can be covered by makeup.

Injection therapy can sometimes make the treatment worse than the problem, especially if a pigment stain occurs at the injection site. This is a poor trade-off, especially when the only purpose in injecting the spider veins is a cosmetic one.

•• NOTHING BETTER THAN SOMETHING

Q. *Many exercise classes seem to operate under the idea that "something is better than nothing," that almost any type of movement is better than just sitting at home watching television. Is this concept correct?*

A. Arthur Jones, founder of Nautilus Sports/Medical Industries, recently addressed the Florida Physical Education Association's annual meeting in Orlando. He estimated that if everyone in the United States realistically rated their physical fitness experiences throughout their lifetime, on a scale from −10 to +10, the combined overall average would be −4. In other words, physical fitness activities have caused more harm than good. He also stated that if everyone in the United States suddenly stopped participating in all fitness activities, the health of the nation would significantly improve in a matter of weeks, because their physical fitness experiences would rise from −4 to something closer to 0.

Although the above is an opinion and not a proven fact, national medical records do reveal that each year sport and fitness activities are responsible for 20 million accidents serious enough to require the attention of a doctor.

The above data reveal that there are serious problems with the physical fitness situation in the United States. Much of this is a result of the proliferation of fitness frauds and easy-exercise methods.

It is unfortunate when "nothing is better than something" may be more appropriate than "something is better than nothing."

Exercise should prevent injury, not cause it. Exercise should improve health, not erode it. Super-slow exercise will accomplish these goals in a fast, efficient manner.

•• EXERCISING DURING ILLNESS

Q. *What about performing the recommended exercise routines when I don't feel well?*

A. Don't try to practice intense exercise when ill. Both high-intensity exercise and illness make heavy demands on your recovery ability. Illnesses can interfere with recovery from strenuous exercise, and strenuous exercise can aggravate some illnesses.

As a rule, you should rest one day for every day you are sick before resuming your strength-training program. When you start exercising again, you should lower the intensity slightly for several workouts.

•• SWEATING AND FAT LOSS

Q. *Will working up a good sweat during exercising help me in losing fat?*

A. Sweating does not help you reduce body fat, although it may temporarily reduce your weight. Weight loss from working up a sweat stems from depletion of water, not fat. As soon as you quench your thirst, your weight usually returns to normal.

Excessive sweating can cause your body to start preserving fat. You should particularly avoid rubber sweat suits, belts, and wraps. Even steam, sauna, and whirlpool baths can lead to problems.

Ideally you should exercise in a cool environment. A temperature between 65 and 70 degrees Fahrenheit is desirable.

•• WHIRLPOOLS

Q. *Are there any fitness benefits from soaking in a whirlpool bath for 5 to 10 minutes after a hard workout?*

A. Physicians and therapists often recommend whirlpool therapy for people with certain muscle, tendon, and ligament injuries. From a physical fitness rather than rehabilitation viewpoint, however, there are no beneficial effects from soaking in a whirlpool. There are, in fact, several good reasons why a fitness-minded person should avoid using one.

First is the problem of heat dissipation. Once a person's body temperature rises above 100 degrees Fahrenheit, serious things begin to happen. The temperature gauges on many whirlpool baths are set at 102 degrees and above, which drastically increases the danger of fainting in the water. Dr. Lawrence Lamb, editor of the *Health Letter,* says there is no reason why the temperature of the water should be above body temperature (98.6 degrees Fahrenheit).

Second, there is the danger of infection from unsanitary water. Warm water has a stimulating effect on the urinary bladder, and we all know what often results. Infection can also spread from fecal matter, genital problems, boils, open sores, and wounds. Furthermore, the warm water of a whirlpool makes an excellent breeding environment for many bacteria. Realizing these facts, physical therapists who use whirlpools in their rehabilitation work are careful to drain the water and scrub the tub after each patient uses it. The standard procedure in many fitness centers is to clean the whirlpool nightly and to drain and replace water weekly.

Third, excessive heat from a whirlpool, sauna, or steam bath can lead to dehydration. Both excessive heat and dehydration are perceived by your body as major stressors. When your body is under major stress it has a tendency to actually preserve your fatty deposits. Your body wants to feel secure, not threatened.

Stay clear of whirlpools and other forms of excessive heat for the duration of the program. Do not let your body get dehydrated. Remember, drinking from 1 to 1 5/8 gallons of water each day will facilitate the fat-loss process.

•• SUPER SLOW

Q. *Isn't this super-slow style of exercise that you recommend a major stressor? Why wouldn't it also cause your body to preserve fat?*

A. Yes, super-slow exercise is a major stressor. If you do too much of it, your body will start preserving fat. The key is to keep the exercise very brief and very intense.

Intense, brief exercise is the most efficient way to stimulate your muscles to grow larger and stronger. Muscular growth is perhaps the foremost priority of the human body.

When you embark on a reduced-calorie diet, your body perceives that something is wrong. It starts preserving fat, as preserving fat is part of your survival mechanism. To prevent this from occurring, you'll need to overrule your survival mechanism by stimulating your muscles to grow. Your muscles will then pull calories from your fat cells to assure their growth. This guarantees that your weight loss will be entirely from fat.

Once again, the exercise itself must be intense and brief. That's why on the Hot Hips and Fabulous Thighs program you only do 8 to 11 exercises per workout. Each workout lasts less than 30 minutes and is repeated only three times per week.

Properly performed, super-slow exercise is the ideal complement to a descending-calorie diet.

Together, they make it possible for you to get the hips and thighs you've always wanted.

···**33**···
Hot Hips and Fabulous Thighs—Forever!

If you combine the ingredients of this book, there's no reason why you can't have Hot Hips and Fabulous Thighs for life.

You have much to look forward to.

You're going to know how to eat and how to exercise properly under almost any circumstance.

You're going to feel stronger, more energetic, and more alive.

You're going to look terrific. With your new body, you're going to enjoy shopping for clothes—even swimsuits and evening dresses—and you'll wear them with pride.

Losing fat and building muscle will free you from the cocoon of your own self-consciousness so you can be more caring and more giving to others.

You'll be eager to get out in the world, to meet new people, to participate in activities you may never have considered before.

The synergy of it all will increase self-confidence and happiness.

That's what the Hot Hips and Fabulous Thighs program can do for you!

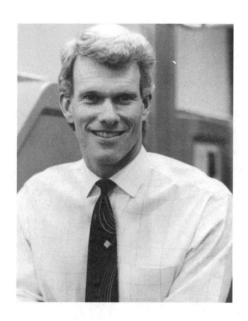

ABOUT THE AUTHOR
• • •

Ellington Darden has a goal: to help people live leaner and stronger longer. For the last twenty years he has worked with thousands of men and women who are seeking ways to improve their self-esteem, feel better physically, look more attractive, and gain results in improved health that can only be achieved through a disciplined approach to nutrition and exercise.

Dr. Darden has been director of research for Nautilus Sports/ Medical Industries since 1973. He holds bachelor's and master's degrees in physical education from Baylor University, and a doctor's degree in exercise science from Florida State University. Two years of post-doctoral study in food and nutrition set him on the trail that led to this book, which is the outgrowth of five years of research.

Dr. Darden is the author of 34 books. Recent titles include *How to Lose Body Fat, The Nautilus Diet, The Six-Week Fat-to-Muscle Makeover,* and *32 Days to a 32-Inch Waist.* In addition he writes a popular weekly column that appears in the *Dallas Times Herald.* Dr. Darden's contributions were recognized in 1989 when he was honored as one of the top ten health leaders in the United States by the President's Council on Physical Fitness and Sports.

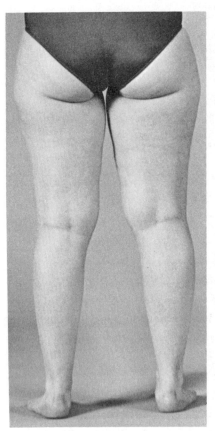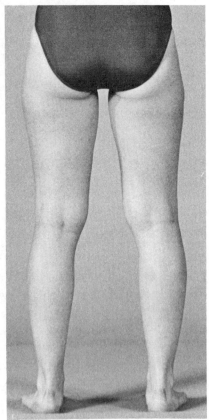

Before   **After**

It took Patti Beran twenty weeks to accomplish this remarkable
metamorphosis. In the process she lost 8 1/8 inches off her hips and
9 1/4 inches off her upper thighs.